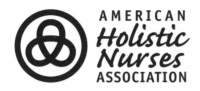

AMERICAN
Holistic
Nurses
ASSOCIATION

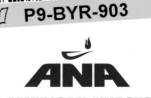

AMERICAN NURSES
ASSOCIATION

HOLISTIC NURSING:
SCOPE AND STANDARDS
OF PRACTICE

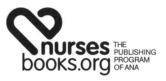

nurses THE
PUBLISHING
books.org PROGRAM
OF ANA

AMERICAN HOLISTIC NURSES ASSOCIATION
AMERICAN NURSES ASSOCIATION
SILVER SPRING, MARYLAND
2007

Library of Congress Cataloging-in-Publication data

Holistic nursing : scope and standards of practice / American Holistic Nurses Association.
   p. ; cm.
   Includes bibliographical references.
   ISBN-13: 978-1-55810-248-4 (pbk.)
   ISBN-10: 1-55810-248-5 (pbk.)
   1. Holistic nursing—Standards. 2. Holistic nursing. I. American Holistic Nurses
Association. II. American Nurses Association.
   [DNLM: 1. Holistic Nursing–methods. 2. Holistic Nursing–standards.
WY 86.5 H7327 2007]

RT42.H6558 2007
   610.73—dc22
                                         2007006845

The American Nurses Association (ANA) is a national professional association. This ANA publication— *Holistic Nursing: Scope and Standards of Practice*—reflects the thinking of the nursing profession on various issues and should be reviewed in conjunction with state board of nursing policies and practices. State law, rules, and regulations govern the practice of nursing, while *Holistic Nursing: Scope and Standards of Practice* guides nurses in the application of their professional skills and responsibilities.

The American Holistic Nurses Association (AHNA) is a non-profit membership organization that is open to nurses and other individuals interested in holistically oriented health care practices throughout the United States and the world. AHNA is the definitive voice for holistic nursing and supports the education of nurses, allied health practitioners, and the general public on health-related issues and the concepts of holism: a state of harmony among body, mind, emotions and spirit within an ever-changing environment. http://www.ahna.org/

Published by Nursesbooks.org
The Publishing Program of ANA
www.Nursesbooks.org

American Nurses Association
8515 Georgia Avenue, Suite 400
Silver Spring, MD 20910-3492
1-800-274-4ANA
www.Nursingworld.org

The American Nurses Association (ANA) is the only full-service professional organization representing the interests of the nation's 3.1 million registered nurses through its constituent/state nurses associations and its organizational affiliates. The ANA advances the nursing profession by fostering high standards of nursing practice, promoting the rights of nurses in the workplace, projecting a positive and realistic view of nursing, and by lobbying the Congress and regulatory agencies on healthcare issues affecting nurses and the public.

Design: Scott Bell, Arlington, VA; Freedom by Design, Alexandria, VA; Stacy McGuire, Sterling, VA ~ *Composition*: House of Equations, Inc., Arden, NC ~ *Editing*: Lisa Munsat Anthony, Chapel Hill, NC ~ *Printing*: Harris LithoGraphics, Landover, MD.

First printing, May 2007.   Second Printing, April 2010.   Third Printing, March 2011.

ISBN: 978-1-55810-248-4   SAN: 851-3481
1.5M   03/11R

CONTRIBUTORS

Primary contributor:
Carla Mariano, EdD, RN, AHN-BC, FAAIM

The works of many provided the foundation for *Holistic Nursing: Scope and Standards of Practice* (2006). These are cited in the bibliography and in Appendices B, C, and D. Most notably are:

Barbara Montgomery Dossey, PhD, RN, AHN-BC, FAAN
Charlotte Eliopoulos, PhD, RN, MPH, ND
Noreen Cavan Frisch, PhD, AHN-BC, FAAN
Cathi E. Guzzetta, PhD, RN, AHN-BC, FAAN
Lynn Keegan, PhD, RN, AHN-BC, FAAN
Carla Mariano, EdD, RN, AHN-BC, FAAIM
Jean Watson, PhD, RN, AHN-BC, FAAN

The Task Forces and Review Committees for these documents:

- *Standards of Holistic Nursing Practice* (AHNA 2005, revised)

- *Standards of Advanced Holistic Practice for Graduate-Prepared Nurses* (AHNA 2005, revised)

- AHNA Position Statements

Without these invaluable resources and the efforts of numerous holistic nurses throughout the years, this document would not have become a reality.

*****

Sincere and heartfelt appreciation to the following individuals for all of their efforts in bringing this document to fruition, thereby enabling holistic nursing to be recognized as a specialty:

- Deanna Deyo, BFA, MA
  Administrative Assistant
  College of Nursing
  New York University

  Thank you for your editorial expertise, and your remarkable patience and good humor throughout the many iterations of this document.

- Carol Bickford, PhD, RN-BC
  Senior Policy Fellow
  American Nurses Association

  Thank you for your wise and helpful suggestions in the sculpting of this document, your support during the process, and your belief in holistic nursing.

- The Leadership Council and Staff of the American Holistic Nurses Association (AHNA)

- Charlotte McGuire and the founding members of the AHNA

  Thank you for your encouragement and unending conviction that holistic nursing would eventually become a specialty.

ANA Staff

Carol J. Bickford, PhD, RN,BC—Content editor
Yvonne Daley Humes, MSA—Project coordinator
Matthew Seiler, RN, Esq.—Legal counsel

Winifred Carson-Smith, JD—Legal consultant

CONTENTS

Introduction: Overview of the Scope and Standards of Holistic Nursing

Extraordinary changes have occurred in health care and nursing during the past decade. The purpose of this document is to articulate the scope and standards of the specialty practice of holistic nursing and to inform holistic nurses, the nursing profession, other healthcare providers and disciplines, employers, third-party payers, legislators, and the public about the unique scope of knowledge and the standards of practice and professional performance of a holistic nurse.

Function of the Scope of Practice Statement of Holistic Nursing

The scope of practice statement describes the *who, what, where, when, why*, and *how* of the practice of holistic nursing. The answers to these questions provide a picture of that specialty nursing practice, its boundaries, and its membership.

Nursing: Scope and Standards of Practice (ANA 2004) applies to all professional registered nurses engaged in practice, regardless of specialty, practice setting, or educational preparation. With the *Code of Ethics for Nurses with Interpretive Statements* (ANA 2001) and *Nursing's Social Policy Statement, Second Edition* (ANA 2003), it forms the foundation of practice for all registered nurses. The scope of holistic nursing practice is specific to this specialty, but it builds on the scope of practice expected of all registered nurses.

Function of the Standards of Holistic Nursing

"Standards are authoritative statements by which the nursing profession describes the responsibilities for which its practitioners are accountable. Consequently, standards reflect the values and priorities of the profession. Standards provide direction for professional nursing practice and a framework for evaluation of this practice. Written in measurable terms, these standards define the nursing profession's accountability to the public and the outcomes for which registered nurses are responsible" (ANA 2004, p. 1). The standards of holistic nursing practice are specific to this specialty, but build on the standards of practice expected of all registered nurses.

Development of the Original Holistic Nursing Standards of Practice: Basic and Advanced

Basic Standards Development

The American Holistic Nurses Association (AHNA) first developed *Standards of Holistic Nursing Practice* in 1990, which were revised in 1995. Between 1994 and 1997, the AHNA conducted a three-year role delineation study, the Inventory of Professional Activities and Knowledge of a Holistic Nurse (IPAKHN Survey). In this practice analysis study the activities and knowledge basic to current holistic nursing practice were determined through administration of a structured inventory to a representative sample of holistic nurses.

This three-year endeavor was successfully completed by a four-member AHNA Task Force and reviewed by the AHNA Leadership Council, select AHNA members, and other recognized holistic nurse members and nonmembers, representing the diversity of holistic nurse representation from practice, education, research, and administration.

An extensive five-step process was used to revise the 1995 *AHNA Standards of Holistic Nursing Practice* and to delineate core values.

Step 1: Literature Review, Inventory of Professional Activities and Knowledge of a Holistic Nurse (IPAKHN) Survey Data Analysis, and Expert Reviews

The (IPAKHN) Survey was created after an extensive literature review of the *Journal of Holistic Nursing* (1985–1995), *Holistic Nursing Practice* (1985–1995), and numerous other holistic nursing journals, holistic-related books, and research. The Task Force reviewed these same journals from 1996–1998 as well as *Essential Readings in Holistic Nursing* (Guzzetta 1998) as a basis for the latest revisions. The eight-member AHNA Standards of Practice Task Force Committee used as a foundation the IPAKHN Survey data analysis recommendations.

In early 1998, the AHNA Standards of Practice Task Force also announced the process in *Beginnings*, the newsletter of AHNA, thus involving the AHNA membership and other recognized holistic nurse experts. Following this announcement, significant suggestions were submitted to the AHNA Task Force.

Step 2: Review Process

Following Step 1, the AHNA Standards of Practice Task Force Committee incorporated the suggestions and additional data from the literature review and the IPAKHN Survey Analysis that reflected the most recent holistic nursing professional activities, knowledge, and caring–healing modalities. Based on this review and the additional comments, deletions, modifications, and recommendations by expert nurses, five areas were further refined and developed:

- The AHNA holistic nursing description was expanded.
- Guidelines were stated for better utilization and integration of the Standards in clinical practice, education, and research.
- Interventions most frequently used in holistic nursing practice were identified based on the IPAKHN Survey data analysis.
- Holistic nursing practice definitions were identified and described.
- A summary page of five Core Value statements was developed.

The five Core Values were followed by Standards of Practice to reflect the dynamic art and science of holistic nursing practice.

Step 3: AHNA Standards of Practice Advisory Committee

Following Step 2, the revised AHNA Standards of Practice were next sent to the 24-member Advisory Committee, who gave additional comments, modifications, and recommendations. Step 3 involved five subsequent revision rounds by the AHNA Task Force Committee before consensus was achieved. It was again sent to the Advisory Committee for additional comments, modifications, and recommendations, which were incorporated.

Step 4: AHNA Standards of Practice Review Committee

Following Step 3, the revised AHNA Standards of Practice were next sent to the 24-member Review Committee, who gave additional comments, deletions, modifications, and recommendations. Step 4 involved three subsequent revision rounds by the AHNA Task Force Committee before consensus was achieved. It was again sent to the Review Committee for additional comments, deletions, modifications, and recommendations, which were incorporated.

The second phase of Step 4 involved a review by a ten-member AHNA Leadership Council, who gave additional comments, deletions, modifications, and recommendations. Step 4 involved only one round by the AHNA Task Force Committee before consensus was achieved. Following the revision process fourth round of responses from the AHNA Task Force Committee, the Advisory Committee, the Review Committee, and the Leadership Committee, consensus on the revised *Standards of Holistic Nursing Practice* (AHNA) was achieved.

Step 5: AHNA Standards of Practice Leadership Council

Following Step 4, the final draft of the *Standards of Holistic Nursing Practice* was submitted to the AHNA Leadership Council prior to the June 1999 AHNA Board meeting. After discussion, a final vote of approval accepted the *Standards of Holistic Nursing Practice*. These were then presented at the annual AHNA Conference June 1999 AHNA Business Meeting in Scottsdale, Arizona. The AHNA Standards received a vote of approval by the AHNA membership. Minor editorial changes were approved by the AHNA Leadership Council in January 2000, with additional minor revisions in 2004 and 2005. (Adapted from Frisch et al. 2000, with permission from the publisher.)

The 2005 *Standards of Holistic Nursing Practice* (AHNA) contained the following five core values.

- Core Value 1. Holistic Philosophy, Theories, and Ethics
- Core Value 2. Holistic Caring Process
- Core Value 3. Holistic Communication, Therapeutic Environment, and Cultural Diversity
- Core Value 4. Holistic Education and Research
- Core Value 5. Holistic Nurse Self-Care

Advanced Standards Development

In response to the growing number of graduate programs with a holistic nursing focus, the AHNA Leadership Council appointed a nine-member task force in January 2000 to develop standards for advanced practice. From that time until October 2001, the Task Force worked to develop standards for advanced holistic nursing practice. The final draft was completed and accepted for submission to the Council by the Task Force Members in September 2001.

The Task Force used the Core Values as the foundation for developing the advanced practice standards. Regardless of the type of practice of the holistic nurse, these values should serve as the philosophical underpinning for practice. *The Essentials of Master's Education for Advanced Practice Nursing* (1996), published by the American Association of Colleges of Nursing, and ANA's *Scope and Standards of Advanced Practice Registered*

Nursing Practice (1996) served as additional guides for the scope of practice that should be addressed by the standards, since these documents are employed in the development of graduate nursing curricula.

AHNA conducted an advanced practice standards review process similar to that used to create the basic practice standards. In addition to the Task Force, leaders in the field of holistic nursing and nursing education were asked to review the draft standards to establish content validity. These leaders were to form the Responding Committee, and their purpose would be to make sure the standards would be congruent with national developments in graduate nursing education and holistic theory development. Over the Spring, seven national holistic nursing leaders were identified, and they agreed to serve in this way. In July/ August 2000 a call went out to the general membership asking for graduate-prepared holistic nurses to become members of a Corresponding Committee. The purpose of this committee was to review the 2000 standards and provide valuable input regarding actual practice. Eleven people completed the Corresponding Committee process.

Draft 1 was completed and circulated to Task Force members for review and comment in Spring 2000. The comments were then used to prepare Draft 2 for the Task Force to review. A decision was made that the standards for advanced practice would apply to those nurses with a graduate degree even though there are nurses in practice with an expanded scope created not by graduate education but by certifications in particular specialties. These certifications were created before graduate education became the entry level for advanced practice. It was felt that the basic standards more than adequately address the scope of practice for all except graduate practice, and the need was to have standards to address holistic nursing practice by graduate-prepared nurses that would guide in the development of curricula for graduate education in holistic nursing.

Draft 3 was completed during the Summer of 2000 and then circulated in the Fall to Task Force members. Draft 4 was prepared from the feedback of Task Force members and circulated to the Responding and Corresponding Committees for review and comment. This draft was distributed to all Task Force and Committee Members in March 2001.

Comments on Draft 4 were received throughout the Spring and Summer of 2001. In September these comments were collated into a final draft. Draft 5, the final draft, was reviewed and accepted for submission to the Leadership Council. The *Standards of Advanced Holistic Nursing Practice for Graduate-Prepared Nurses* were approved and adopted by the AHNA Leadership Council in January 2002, followed by a minor revision in 2005. (Adapted from *Standards of Advanced Holistic Nursing Practice for Graduate-Prepared Nurses,* AHNA 2005.)

During the interval from 2004 until 2006 the original *Standards of Holistic Nursing Practice* (Advanced and Basic) were substantively revised to incorporate language and content required by ANA to support the application for formal recognition of Holistic Nursing as a nursing specialty. The Leadership Council of the AHNA reviewed and approved the preliminary draft statement of *Standards* in June 2005, and then the draft *Holistic Nursing: Scope and Standards of Practice* in March 2006.

Summary

Holistic Nursing: Scope and Standards of Practice (2007) reflects a consensus and provides a blueprint for holistic practice, education, and research. These *Standards* guide clinicians, educators, researchers, nurse managers, and administrators in professional activities, knowledge, and performance that are relevant to holistic nursing basic and advanced practice, education, research, and management.

Holistic Nursing:
Scope of Practice

Definition and Overview of Holistic Nursing

Holistic nursing is defined as "all nursing practice that has healing the whole person as its goal" (AHNA 1998).

Holistic nursing embraces all nursing that has the enhancement of healing the whole person from birth to death—and all age groups from infant to elder—as its goal. Holistic nursing recognizes that there are two views regarding holism: that holism involves identifying the interrelationships of the bio-psycho-social-spiritual dimensions of the person, recognizing that the whole is greater than the sum of its parts; and that holism involves understanding the individual as a unitary whole in mutual process with the environment. Holistic nursing responds to both views, believing that the goals of nursing can be achieved within either framework.

Holistic nursing focuses on protecting, promoting, and optimizing health and wellness, assisting healing, preventing illness and injury, alleviating suffering, and supporting people to find peace, comfort, harmony, and balance through the diagnosis and treatment of human response.

Holistic nursing care is person–relationship centered and healing oriented vs. disease/cure oriented. Holistic nursing emphasizes practices of self-care, intentionality, presence, mindfulness, and therapeutic use of self as pivotal for facilitation of healing and patterning of wellness in others. Holistic nursing is prospective, focusing on:

- Comprehensive health promotion and health risk reduction.
- Proactive interventions that address antecedents and mediators of disease.
- Opportunities in each individual's experiences of illness and disease for the individual's transformation, growth, and finding of meaning.

The holistic nurse is an instrument of healing and a facilitator in the healing process. Holistic nurses honor the individual's subjective experience about health, health beliefs, and values. To become therapeutic partners with individuals, families, communities, and populations, holistic nursing practice draws on nursing knowledge, theories, research, expertise, intuition, and creativity incorporating the roles of clinician, educator, consultant, partner, role model, and advocate. Holistic nursing practice encourages peer review of professional practice in various clinical settings and provides care based on current professional standards, laws, and regulations governing nursing practice.

Holistic nurses integrate complementary/alternative modalities (CAM) into clinical practice to treat people's physiological, psychological, and spiritual needs. Doing so does not negate the validity of conventional medical therapies but serves to complement, broaden, and enrich the scope of nursing practice and to help individuals access their greatest healing potential. Integration rather than separation is advocated.

Practicing holistic nursing requires nurses to integrate self-care, self-responsibility, spirituality, and reflection in their own lives. This leads the nurse to greater awareness of the interconnectedness with oneself, others, nature, and God/LifeForce/Absolute/Transcendent. This awareness further enhances nurses' understanding of all individuals and their relationships to the human and global community, and it permits nurses to use this awareness to facilitate the healing process.

The phenomena of concern to holistic nursing include, but are not limited to:

- The caring-healing relationship
- The subjective experience of and meanings ascribed to health, illness, wellness, healing, birth, growth and development, and dying
- The cultural values and beliefs and folk practices of health, illness, and healing
- Spirituality in nursing care
- The evaluation of complementary/alternative modalities used in nursing practice
- Comprehensive health promotion and disease prevention
- Self-care processes
- Physical, mental, emotional, and spiritual comfort, discomfort, and pain

- Empowerment, decision-making, and the ability to make informed choices
- Social and economic policies and their effects on the health of individuals, families, and communities
- Diverse and alternative healthcare systems and their relationships with access and quality of health care
- The environment and the prevention of disease

This document, used in conjunction with *Nursing's Social Policy Statement, Second Edition* (ANA 2003), *Nursing: Scope and Standards of Practice* (ANA 2004), *Code of Ethics for Nurses with Interpretive Statements* (ANA 2001), and the laws, statutes, and regulations related to nursing practice for their state, commonwealth, or territory, delineates the professional responsibilities of a holistic nurse.

Evolution of Holistic Nursing

"Holism" in health care is a philosophy that emanated directly from Florence Nightingale, who believed in care that focused on unity, wellness, and the interrelationship of human beings, events, and environment. Even Hippocrates, the father of Western medicine, espoused a holistic orientation when he taught doctors to observe their patients' life circumstances and emotional states. Socrates stated, "Curing the soul; that is the first thing." In holism, symptoms are believed to be an expression of the body's wisdom as it reacts to cure its own imbalance or disease.

The root of the word *heal* comes from the Greek word *halos* and the Anglo-Saxon word *healan*, which means "to be or to become whole." The word *holy* also comes from the same source. Healing means "making whole"—or restoring balance and harmony. It is movement toward a sense of wholeness and completion. Healing therefore is the integration of the totality of the person in body, mind, emotion, spirit, and environment.

One of the driving forces behind the holistic nursing movement in the United States was the formation of the American Holistic Nurses Association (AHNA). In 1980, founder Charlotte McGuire and 75 founding members began the national organization in Houston, Texas. The national office is now located in Flagstaff, Arizona. AHNA has as its mission to unite nurses in healing with a focus on holistic principles of health, preventive education, and the integration of allopathic and complementary caring–healing modalities to facilitate care of the whole person and significant others. From its inception in 1980, the American Holistic Nurses Association (AHNA) has been the leader in developing and advancing holistic principles, practices, and guidelines. The Association predicted that holistic principles, caring–healing, and the integration of complementary/alternative therapies would emerge into mainstream health care.

The AHNA, the definitive voice for holistic nursing, is committed to promoting wholeness and wellness in individuals/families/communities, nurses themselves, the nursing profession, and the environment. Through its various activities, the AHNA provides vision, direction, and leadership in the advancement of holistic nursing; integrates the art and science of nursing in the profession; empowers holistic nursing through education, research, and standards; encourages nurses to be models of wellness; honors individual excellence in the advancement of holistic nursing; and influences policy to change the healthcare system to a more humanistic orientation.

The goals and endeavors of the AHNA have continued to map conceptual frameworks and the blueprint for holistic nursing practice, education, and research, which is the most complete way to conceptualize and practice professional nursing. Beginning in 1993, AHNA undertook an organization development process that included the following areas:

- Identification of the steps toward national certification in 1993–1994

- Revision of the 1990 *Standards of Holistic Nursing Practice*, completed in 1995

- Completing a role delineation study, the *Inventory of Professional Activities and Knowledge Statements of a Holistic Nurse* (also known as the IPAKHN Survey) in 1997

- Developing a national Holistic Nursing Certification Examination, completed in 1997

- Completing major revisions of the 1995 *Standards of Holistic Nursing Practice* in 1999, with additional editorial changes in January 2000 and 2005

- Developing a Core Curriculum for basic holistic nursing based on the Basic Standards (1997)
- Approving and adopting *Standards of Advanced Holistic Nursing Practice for Graduate-Prepared Nurses* (2002, revised 2005)
- Developing a Core Curriculum for advanced holistic nursing based on the Advanced Standards (2003)
- Developing the Certification Exam for Advanced Holistic Nursing Practice by The American Holistic Nurses Certification Corporation (AHNCC) in 2004. This exam was first offered in March 2005.
- Revising the 2004 basic and advanced *Standards of Holistic Nursing Practice* to meet ANA criteria for recognition of holistic nursing as a specialty

Other AHNA activities that support and promote holistic nursing include:

- Collaborating with other organizations to strengthen the voice of nursing
- Endorsing certificate programs for nurses that have content in holistic nursing and/or complementary/alternative healing modalities
- Organizing networking groups to further holistic nursing
- Providing and approving continuing education programs featuring holistic health topics, holistic research, and holistic education
- Granting awards for holistic nursing research
- Publishing several informational, educational, research, and professional support materials
- Sponsoring the World-Wide Commemorative Moment for Florence Nightingale and Nursing
- Offering the National Student Sponsorship Initiative

There are now increasing numbers of holistic nurses who hold leadership roles as clinicians, educators, authors, and researchers in university-based schools of nursing, practice environments, nursing, and other professional organizations.

Membership in the AHNA is open to all individuals who support the mission of the organization. AHNA's philosophy is that holistic nursing is the *heart* of nursing and the *science* of holism.

Principles of Holistic Nursing

The following principles—Person, Healing/Health, Practice—underlie holistic nursing:

Person

- There is unity, totality, and connectedness of everyone and everything (body, mind, emotion, spirit, sexuality, age, environment, social/cultural, belief systems, relationships, context).

- Human beings are unique and inherently good.

- People are able to find meaning and purpose in their own life, experiences, and illness.

- All people have an innate power and capacity for self healing. Health/illness is subjectively described and determined by the view of the individual. Therefore, the person is honored in all phases of his/her healing process regardless of expectations or outcomes.

- People/persons/individuals are the recipients of holistic nursing services. These can be clients, patients, families, significant others, populations, or communities. They may be ill and within the health-care delivery system or well, moving toward personal betterment to enhance well-being.

Healing/Health

- Health and illness are natural and a part of life, learning, and movement toward change and development.

- Health is seen as balance, integration, harmony, right relationship, and the betterment of well-being, not just the absence of disease. Healing can take place without cure. The focus is on health promotion/disease prevention/health restoration/lifestyle patterns and habits, as well as symptom relief.

- Illness is considered a teacher and an opportunity for self-awareness and growth as part of the life process. Symptoms are respected as messages.

- People as active partners in the healing process are empowered when they take some control of their own lives, health, and well-being including personal choices and relationships.

- Treatment is a process that considers the root of the problem, not merely treating the obvious signs and symptoms.

Practice

- Practice is a science (critical thinking, reflection, evidence/research/ theory as underlying practice) and an art (intuition, creativity, presence, self/personal knowing as integral to practice).
- The values and ethic of holism, caring, moral insight, dignity, integrity, competence, responsibility, accountability, and legality underlie holistic nursing practice.
- There are various philosophies and paradigms of health, illness, healing, and approaches/models for the delivery of health care, both in the U.S. and in other cultures, that need to be understood and utilized.
- Older adults represent the predominant population served by nurses.
- Public policy and the healthcare delivery system influence the health and well-being of society and professional nursing.

Nursing Roles

- Using warmth, compassion, caring, authenticity, respect, trust, and relationship as instruments of healing in and of themselves, as part of the healing environment.
- Using conventional nursing interventions as well as holistic/ complementary/alternative/integrative modalities that enhance the body-mind-emotion-spirit-environment connectedness to foster healing, health, wholeness, and well-being of people.
- Collaborating and partnering with all constituencies in the health process including the person receiving care and family, community, peers, and other disciplines. Using principles and skills of cooperation, alliance, and respect and honoring the contributions of all.
- Participating in the change process to develop more caring cultures in which to practice and learn.
- Assisting nurses to nurture and heal themselves.

- Participating in activities that contribute to the improvement of communities and the environment and to the betterment of public health.

- Acting as an advocate for the rights of and equitable distribution and access to health care for all persons, especially vulnerable populations.

- Honoring the ecosystem and our relationship with and need to preserve it, as we are all connected.

Self-Care

- The nurse's self-reflection and self-assessment, self-care, healing, and personal development are necessary for service to others and growth/change in one's own well-being and understanding of one's own personal journey.

- The nurse values oneself and one's calling to holistic nursing as a life purpose.

Integrating the Art and Science of Nursing: Core Values

The art and science of holistic nursing emanates from these five core values, which are described in this section:

- Core Value 1. Holistic Philosophy, Theories, and Ethics

- Core Value 2. Holistic Caring Process

- Core Value 3. Holistic Communication, Therapeutic Environment, and Cultural Diversity

- Core Value 4. Holistic Education and Research

- Core Value 5. Holistic Nurse Self-Care

Core Value 1. Holistic Philosophy, Theories, and Ethics

Holistic nurses recognize the human health experience as a complicated, dynamic relationship of health, illness, and wellness, and they value healing as the desired outcome of the practice of nursing. Their practice is based on scientific foundations (theory, research, evidence-based practice, critical thinking, reflection) and art (relationship, communication, creativity, presence, caring).

Holistic nursing is grounded in nursing knowledge and skill and guided by nursing theory. Florence Nightingale's writings are often referenced as a significant precursor for the development of holistic nursing practice. While each holistic nurse chooses which nursing theory to apply in any individual case, the nursing theories of Jean Watson (Theory of Human Caring), Martha Rogers (the Science of Unitary Human Beings), Margaret Newman (Health as Expanding Consciousness), Madeleine Leininger (Theory of Cultural Care), Rosemarie Rizzo Parse (Theory of Human Becoming), Paterson and Zderad (Humanistic Nursing Theory), and Helen Erickson (Modeling and Role-Modeling) are most frequently used to support holistic nursing practice.

In addition to nursing theory, holistic nurses utilize other theories and perspectives of wholeness and healing that guide their practice. These scientific theories and philosophies present a worldview of connectedness, e.g., theories of consciousness; energy field theory; Carl Pribram's Holographic Universe; David Bohm's Implicate/Explicate Order; Candace Pert's psychoneuroimmunology; Rupert Sheldrake's morphogenic fields; Ken Wilbur's Spectrum of Consciousness and Integral Psychology; Pierre Tielhard de Chardin's philosophy; spirituality; and alternative medical systems such as traditional Oriental medicine, Ayurveda, Native American and indigenous healing, and Eastern contemplative orientations such as Zen and Taoism.

Holistic nurses further recognize and honor the ethic that the person is the authority on his or her own health experience. The holistic nurse is an "option giver," i.e., helping the person develop an understanding of alternatives and implications of various health and treatment options.

The holistic nurse first ascertains what the individual thinks or believes is happening to them and then assists the person to identify what will help his/her situation. The assessment begins from where the individual is. The holistic nurse then discusses options, including the person's choices, across a continuum, including possible effects and implications of each. For instance, if a person diagnosed with cancer is experiencing nausea due to chemotherapy, the individual and nurse may discuss the choices and effects of pharmacologic agents, imagery, homeopathic remedies, etc., or a combination of these. The holistic nurse acts as partner and co-prescriptor vs. sole prescriber. The relationship is a co-piloting of the individual's health experience in which the nurse respects the person's decision about his or her own health. It is a process of engagement rather than compliance.

Client narratives, whether they arise from individuals, families, or communities, provide the context of the experiences and are used as an important focus in understanding the person's situation. Holistic nurses hold the belief that people, through their inherent capacities, heal themselves. Therefore, the holistic nurse is not the healer but the guide and facilitator of the individual's own healing.

In the belief that all things are connected, the holistic perspective espouses that an individual's actions have a ripple effect throughout humanity. Holism places the greatest worth on individuals' developing higher levels of human awareness. This, in turn, elevates the whole of humanity. Holistic nurses believe in the sacredness of one's self and of all nature. One's inner self and the collective greater self have stewardship not only over one's body, mind, and spirit, but also over our planet. Holistic nurses focus on the meaning and quality of life deriving from their own character and from their relationship to the universe rather than imposed from without.

Holistic nurses hold to a professional ethic of caring and healing that seeks to preserve wholeness and dignity of self and others. They support human dignity by advocating and adhering to *The Patient's Bill of Rights in Medicare and Medicaid* (U.S. DHHS 1999a), ANA's *Code of Ethics for Nurses with Interpretive Standards* (2001), and AHNA's *Position Statement on Holistic Nursing Ethics* (2007), the latter of which is included in Appendix D (page 120).

Core Value 2. Holistic Caring Process

Holistic nurses provide care that recognizes the totality of the human being (the interconnectedness of body, mind, emotion, spirit, social/cultural, relationship, context, and environment). This is an integrated as well as comprehensive approach. While physical symptoms are being treated, a holistic nurse would also focus on how the individual is cognitively perceiving and emotionally dealing with the illness; its effect on the person's family and social relationships and economic resources; the person's values and cultural, spiritual beliefs and preferences regarding treatment; and the meaning of this experience to the person's life. But in addition, a holistic nurse may also incorporate a number of alternative modalities (e.g., cognitive restructuring, stress management, visualization and imagery, hypnotherapy, aromatherapy, Therapeutic Touch, Healing Touch) with conventional nursing interventions. Holistic nurses focus on care interventions that promote healing, peace, comfort, and a subjective sense of well-being for the person.

The holistic caring process involves six often simultaneously occurring steps: assessment, diagnosis (identification of pattern/problem/need/health issue), outcomes, therapeutic plan of care, implementation, and evaluation. Holistic nurses apply the holistic caring process with individuals or families across the lifespan, population groups, and communities, and in all settings.

Holistic nurses incorporate a variety of roles in their practice, including expert clinician and facilitator of healing; consultant and collaborator; educator and guide; administrator, leader, and change agent; researcher; and advocate. They strongly emphasize partnership with individuals throughout the entire decision-making process.

Holistic assessments include not only the physical, functional, psychosocial, mental, emotional, cultural, and sexual aspects, but also the spiritual, transpersonal, and energy field assessments of the whole person. Energy assessments are based on the concept that all beings are composed of energy. Congestion or stagnation of energy in any realm creates dis-harmony and dis-ease. Spiritual assessments glean not only religious beliefs and practices but also query about a person's meaning and purpose in life and how that may have changed due to the present health experience. Spiritual assessments also include questions about an individual's sense of serenity and peace, what provides joy and fulfillment, and the source of strength and hope.

Holistic assessment data are interpreted into patterns/challenges/needs from which meaning and understanding of the health/disease experience can be mutually identified with the person. An important responsibility is that of helping the person to identify risk factors such as lifestyle, habits, beliefs and values, personal and family health history, and age-related conditions that influence health and then to utilize opportunities to increase well-being. The focus is on the individual's goals, not the nurse's goals.

Therapeutic plans of care respect the person's experience and the uniqueness of each healing journey. The same illness may have very different manifestations in different individuals. A major aspect of holistic nursing practice, in addition to competence, is intention—that is, intending for the wholeness, well-being, and highest good of the person with every encounter and intervention. This honors and reinforces the innate capacity of people to heal themselves. Therefore, holistic nurses respect that outcomes may not be those expected and may evolve differently based on the person's own individual healing process and health choices. Holistic nurses endeavor to detach themselves from the outcomes. The nurse does not produce the outcomes; the individual's own healing process produces the outcomes, and the nurse facilitates this process. A significant focus is on guiding individuals and significant others to utilize their own inner strength and resources through the course of healing.

Appropriate and evidence-based information (including current knowledge, practice, and research) regarding the health condition and various treatments and therapies and their side effects is consistently provided. Holistic care always occurs within the scope and standards of practice of registered nursing and in accordance with state and federal laws and regulations.

In addition to conventional interventions, holistic nurses have knowledge of and integrate a number of CAM approaches, which have been categorized by the National Center for Complementary and Alternative Medicine (2005). (See also Appendix A.) These include the following categories:

- Whole medical systems, such as Ayurveda, Traditional Oriental Medicine, Homeopathy, Naturopathy, Acupuncture, Native American and Latin American indigenous practices

- Mind–body interventions, such as meditation, relaxation, imagery, hypnosis, yoga, t'ai chi, prayer, art, music and dance therapies, cognitive-behavioral therapy, biofeedback, therapeutic counseling, and stress management

- Biologically based therapies, such as herbal therapies, diet therapies, nutritional supplements, and vitamin and mineral supplements

- Manipulative and body-based methods, such as chiropractic, massage therapy, osteopathy, Rolfing, reflexology, Alexander Technique, and Craniosacral therapy

- Energy therapies, such as Therapeutic Touch, Reiki, Qi Gong, Acupressure, Healing Touch, and magnet therapy

Therapies frequently incorporated in holistic nursing practice include the following interventions listed in the Nursing Interventions Classification (NIC): meditation; relaxation therapy; breath work; music, art, aroma therapies; energy-based touch therapies such as Therapeutic Touch, Healing Touch, Reiki; acupressure; massage; guided imagery; animal-assisted therapy; biofeedback; prayer; reflexology; diet; herbology; and homeopathy. Interventions frequently employed in holistic nursing practice in addition to conventional nursing interventions include: anxiety reduction and stress management, calming technique, emotional support, exercise and nutrition promotion, smoking cessation promotion, patient contracting, resiliency promotion, forgiveness facilitation, hope installation, presence, journaling, counseling, cognitive therapy, self-help, spiritual support, and environmental management.

As many of today's healthcare problems are stress related, holistic nurses empower individuals by teaching them techniques to reduce their stress. Many interventions used in holistic nursing elicit the relaxation response (e.g., breath work, meditation, relaxation, imagery, aromatherapy and use of essential oils, diet). People can learn these therapies and use them without the intervention of a healthcare provider. This allows a person to take an active role in the management of his/her own health care. Holistic nurses also can teach families and caregivers to use these techniques for loved ones who may be ill (e.g., simple foot or hand massage for older clients with dementia). In addition, individuals are taught how to evaluate their own responses to these modalities.

Holistic nurses prescribe as legally authorized. They instruct individuals regarding drug, herbal, and homeopathic regimens and, importantly, the side effects and interactions of these therapies. They consult, collaborate, and refer, as necessary, to both conventional allopathic providers and to holistic practitioners. They provide information and counseling to people about alternative, complementary, integrative, and conventional healthcare practices. Very importantly, holistic nurses facilitate negotiation of services as they guide individuals and families between conventional Western medical and alternative systems. Holistic nurses, in partnership with the individual and others, evaluate if care is effective and if there are changes in the meaning of the health experience for the individual.

Core Value 3. Holistic Communication, Therapeutic Environment, and Cultural Diversity

The holistic nurse's communication ensures that each individual experiences the presence of the nurse as authentic, caring, compassionate, and sincere. This is more than simply using therapeutic techniques such as responding, reflecting, summarizing, etc. This is deep listening or, as some say, "listening with the heart and not just the ears." It is done with conscious intention and without preconceptions, busyness, distractions, or analysis. It takes place in the "now" within an atmosphere of shared humanness, i.e., human being to human being. Through presence or "being with in the moment," holistic nurses provide each person with an interpersonal encounter that is experienced as a connection with one who is giving *undivided* attention to the needs and concerns of the individual. Using unconditional positive regard, holistic nurses convey to the individual receiving care the belief in his or her worth and value as a human being, not solely the recipient of medical and nursing interventions.

The importance of context in understanding the person's health experience is always recognized. Space and time are allowed for exploration. Each person's health encounter is truly seen as unique and may be contrary to conventional knowledge and treatments. Therefore, the holistic nurse must be comfortable with ambiguity, paradox, and uncertainty. This requires a perspective that the nurse is not "the expert" regarding another's health/illness experience.

Holistic nurses have a knowledge base of the use and meanings of symbolic language and use interventions such as imagery, creation of sacred space and personal rituals, dream exploration, and aesthetic therapies such as music, visual arts, and dance. They encourage and support others in the use of prayer, meditation, or other spiritual and symbolic practices for healing purposes.

A cornerstone of holistic nursing practice is assisting individuals to find meaning in their experience. Regardless of the health/illness condition, the meaning that individuals ascribe to their situation can influence their response to it. Holistic nurses attend to the subjective world of the individual. They consider meanings such as the person's concerns in relation to health, family relationships, employment, and economics, as well as to deeper meanings related to the person's purpose in life. Regardless of the technology or treatment, holistic nurses address the human spirit as a major force in healing. The person's perception of meaning is related to all factors in health-wellness-disease-illness.

Holistic nurses realize that suffering, illness, and disease are natural components of the human condition and have the potential to teach about oneself, one's relationships, and the universe. Every experience is valued for its meaning and lesson.

Holistic nurses have a particular obligation to create a therapeutic environment that values holism, caring, social support, and integration of conventional and CAM approaches to healing. They seek to create caring cultures and environments where individuals, both clients and staff, feel connected, supported, and respected. A particular perspective of holistic nursing is the nurse as the "healing environment" and an instrument of healing. Holistic nurses shape the physical environment (e.g., light, fresh air, pleasant sounds or quiet, neatness and order, healing smells, earth elements). They also provide a relationship-focused environment, the creation of sacred space through presence and intention where others can feel safe, can unfold, can explore the dimensions of self in healing.

Culture, beliefs, and values are an inherent component of a holistic approach. Concepts of health and healing are based in culture and often influence people's actions to promote, maintain, and restore health. Culture also may provide an understanding of a person's concept of the illness or disease and appropriate treatment. Holistic nurses possess knowledge and understanding of numerous cultural traditions and healthcare practices from various racial, ethnic, and social backgrounds. However, holistic nurses honor individuals' understanding and articulation of their own cultural values, beliefs, and health practices rather than reliance on stereotypical cultural classifications and descriptions. These understandings then are used to provide culturally competent care that corresponds with the beliefs, values, traditions, and health practices of individuals and families. Holistic nurses ask individuals, "What do I need to know about you culturally in caring for you?"

Holistic healing is a collaborative approach. Holistic nurses take an active role in trying to remove the political and financial barriers to the inclusion of holistic care in the healthcare system.

Of particular importance to holistic nurses is the human connection with the ecology. They actively participate in building an ecosystem that sustains the well-being of all life. This includes raising the public's consciousness about environmental issues and stressors that affect not only the health of people, but also the health of the planet.

Core Value 4. Holistic Education and Research

Holistic nurses possess an understanding of a wide range of cultural norms and healthcare practices/beliefs/values concerning individuals, families, groups, and communities from varied racial ethnic, spiritual, and social backgrounds. This rich knowledge base reflects their formal academic and continuing education preparation and also includes a wide diversity of practices and modalities outside of conventional medicine. Because of this preparation, holistic nurses serve as both educators and advocates and have a significant impact on peoples' understanding of healthcare options and alternatives.

Additionally, holistic nurses provide much-needed information to individuals on health promotion including such topics as healthy lifestyles, risk-reducing behaviors, preventive self-care, stress management, living with changes secondary to illness and treatment, and opportunities to enhance well-being.

Holistic nurses value all the ways of knowing and learning. They individualize learning and appreciate that science, intuition, introspection, creativity, aesthetics, and culture produce different bodies of knowledge and perspectives. They help others to know themselves and access their own inner wisdom to enhance growth, wholeness, and well-being.

Holistic nurses often guide individuals and families in their healthcare decisions, especially regarding conventional allopathic and complementary alternative practices. Therefore, they must be knowledgeable about the best evidence available for both conventional and CAM therapies. In addition to developing evidence-based practice using research, practice guidelines, and expertise, holistic nurses strongly consider the person's values and healthcare practices and beliefs in practice decisions.

Holistic nurses look at alternative philosophies of science and research methods that are compatible with investigations of humanistic and holistic occurrences; that explore the context in which phenomena occur and the meaning of patterns that evolve; and that take into consideration the interactive nature of the body, mind, emotion, spirit, and environment.

Holistic nurses conduct and evaluate research in diverse areas such as:

- Outcome measures of various holistic therapies, e.g., Therapeutic Touch, prayer, aromatherapy
- Instrument development to measure caring behaviors and dimensions; spirituality; self-transcendence; cultural competence, etc.
- Client responses to holistic interventions in health/illness
- Explorations of clients' lived experiences with various health/illness phenomena
- Theory development in healing, caring, intentionality, cultural constructions, empowerment, etc.

Core Value 5. Holistic Nurse Self-Care

Self-care as well as personal awareness of and continuous focus on being an instrument of healing are significant requirements for holistic nurses. Holistic nurses value themselves and mobilize the necessary resources to care for themselves. They endeavor to integrate self-awareness, self-care, and self-healing into their lives by incorporating practices such as self-assessment, meditation, yoga, good nutrition, energy therapies, movement, art, support, and lifelong learning. Holistic nurses honor their unique patterns and the development of the body, the psychological-social-cultural self, the intellectual self, and the spiritual self. Nurses cannot facilitate healing unless they are in the process of healing themselves. Through continuing education, practice, and self-work, holistic nurses develop the skills of authentic and deep self-reflection and introspection to understand themselves and their journey. It is seen as a lifelong process.

Holistic nurses strive to achieve harmony/balance in their own lives and assist others to do the same. They create healing environments for themselves by attending to their own well-being, letting go of self-destructive behaviors and attitudes, and practicing centering and stress reduction techniques. By doing this, holistic nurses serve as role models to others, be they clients, colleagues, or personal contacts.

Settings for Holistic Nursing Practice

Holistic nurses practice in numerous settings, including but not limited to: private practitioner offices; ambulatory, acute, long-term, and home care settings; complementary care centers; women's health centers; hospice palliative care; psychiatric mental health facilities; schools; rehabilitation centers; community nursing organizations; student and employee health clinics; managed care organizations; independent self-employed practice; correctional facilities; professional nursing and healthcare organizations; administration; staff development; and universities and colleges.

Holistic nursing practice also occurs when there is a request for consultation or when holistic nurses advocate for care that promotes health and prevents disease, illness, or disability for individuals, communities, or the environment, e.g., a holistic nurse may choose not to work in a critical care setting but provide consultation regarding self-care or stress management to nurses in that area. Or, holistic nurses may practice in preoperative and recovery rooms instituting a "Prepare for Surgery" program that teaches individuals having surgery meditation and positive affirmation techniques, pre and post surgery, while incorporating a homeopathic regimen for trauma and cell healing. Employment or voluntary participation of holistic nurses also can influence civic activities and the regulatory and legislative arena at the local, state, national, or international level.

As holistic nursing focuses on wellness, wholeness, and development of the whole person, holistic nurses also practice in health enhancement settings such as spas, gyms, and wellness centers.

Because holistic nursing is a worldview, a way of "being" in the world and not just a modality, holistic nurses can practice in any setting and with individuals throughout the life span. As the public increasingly requests holistic/CAM services, holistic nurses will be increasingly in demand and practice in a wider array of settings. Holistic nursing takes place wherever healing occurs.

Educational Preparation for Holistic Nursing

Holistic nurses are registered nurses who are educationally prepared for practice from an approved school of nursing and are licensed to practice in their individual state, commonwealth, or territory. The holistic registered nurse's experience, education, knowledge, and abilities establish the level of competence. This document identifies the scope of practice of holistic nursing and the specific standards and associated measurement criteria of holistic nurses at both the basic and advanced levels. Regardless of the level of practice, all holistic nurses integrate the previously identified five core values.

A registered nurse may prepare for the specialty of holistic nursing in a variety of ways. Educational offerings range from baccalaureate and graduate courses and programs to continuing education programs with extensive contact hours.

Basic Practice Level

The education of all nursing students preparing for RN licensure includes basic content on physiological, psychological, emotional, and some spiritual processes with populations across the life span and conventional nursing care practices within each of these domains. Additionally, basic nursing education incorporates experiences in a variety of clinical/practice settings from acute care to community. However, the educational focus is most frequently on "specialties" often emanating from the biomedical disease model with cure orientation.

In holistic nursing, the individual across the life span is viewed in context as an integrated body, mind, emotion, social, spirit totality, with the emphasis on wholeness, well-being, health promotion, and healing using both conventional and complementary/alternative practices. Because of the lack of intentional focus on integration, unity, and healing, the educational exposure of most nursing students is not adequate preparation for assuming the specialty role of a holistic nurse.

There are currently seven undergraduate programs in the U.S. endorsed by the American Holistic Nurse Certification Corporation (AHNCC) that prepare undergraduate students in holistic nursing. Additionally, there are many schools of nursing offering both graduate and undergraduate courses in "Holistic Nursing." A survey of schools of nursing in the United States (Fenton and Morris 2003) indicated that almost 60% (n=74) of the responding schools (sample n=125 schools) had a definition of holistic nursing in their curricula and were familiar with *Holistic Nursing Core Curriculum* (see Dossey 1997). The majority of the sample (84.8%, n=106) included at least one complementary/alternative modality (e.g., visualization, relaxation) in their curricula. Twenty-six (21%) schools had faculty who were certified in holistic nursing.

Increasingly, schools of nursing are incorporating holistic nursing practices and complementary/alternative modalities into their curricula, responding to consumer use of CAM and consumer demand for health professionals who are knowledgeable about holistic practices.

To be board certified by the AHNCC at the basic holistic nursing level, a nurse is required to have: (1) an active, unrestricted U.S. license; (2) a baccalaureate or higher degree; (3) at least one year of full-time practice or 2,000 hours of part-time practice within the last five years as a holistic nurse or graduation from an AHNCC-endorsed university; (4) a minimum of 48 contact hours of holistic nursing continuing education within the last 2 years.

Advanced Practice Level

As with the basic level, there are a variety of ways (both academic and professional development) in which registered nurses can acquire the additional specialized knowledge and skills that prepare them for practice as an advanced practice holistic nurse. These nurses are expected to have an active, unrestricted U.S. license and to hold a master's or doctoral degree in nursing and demonstrate a greater depth and scope of knowledge, a greater integration of information, increased complexity of skills and interventions, and notable role autonomy. They provide leadership in practice, teaching, research, consultation, advocacy, and/or policy formation in advancing holistic nursing to improve the holistic health of people.

Presently five graduate programs in the United States that prepare master's students with a specialty in holistic nursing are endorsed by the AHNCC. Other graduate nursing programs have courses in holistic or complementary/alternative practices. Current advanced practice nurses (nurse practitioners, clinical nurse specialists, nurse midwives, nurse anesthetists) are increasingly gaining specialized knowledge preparing them as holistic nurses through post-master's degree programs, continuing education offerings, and certificate programs.

To be board certified by the AHNCC at the advanced holistic nursing level, a licensed nurse must have a graduate degree in nursing and a minimum of 48 contact hours in holistic nursing within the last 2 years.

Continuing Education for Basic and Advanced Practice Levels

The American Holistic Nurses Association (AHNA) is a provider and approver of continuing education, recognized by the American Nurses Credentialing Center. Continuing educational programs, workshops, and lectures in holistic nursing and CAM have been popular nationwide, with AHNA or other bodies granting continuing education units.

AHNA endorses certificate programs in specific areas, including Spirituality, Health and Healing, Reflexology, Imagery, Aromatherapy, Healing Touch, AMMA Therapy®, Clinical Nursing Assessment, and Whole Health Education. It also approves continuing education offerings in holistic nursing and offers the AHNA home study course, Foundations of Holistic Nursing. Other programs in distinct therapies such as Acupuncture, Reiki, Homeopathy, massage, imagery, healing arts, holistic health, Oriental Medicine, nutrition, Ayurveda, Therapeutic Touch, Healing Touch, herbology, chiropractic, etc. are given nationally as degrees, certificates, or continuing education programs by centers, specialty organizations, or schools.

Certification in Holistic Nursing

In 1992, a four-phase AHNA Certificate Program in Holistic Nursing began. On program completion, a nurse was awarded a certificate in holistic nursing. In 1994, the AHNA Leadership Council appointed an AHNA Task Force Committee to explore steps toward the development of holistic nursing certification through a national certification examination.

The AHNA Leadership Council appointed an AHNA Certification Committee to serve as the governing body to oversee the process of certification of holistic nurses by examination until a separate certification corporation was established. In 1997, the AHNA Certification Board established a separate 501C-3 organization, the American Holistic Nurses' Certification Corporation (AHNCC), to act as the credentialing body for the Holistic Nursing Certification Examination. The AHNCC now has five directors who are voting members, and two non-voting members, one of whom is the liaison of the AHNA Leadership Council. Of the voting members, one represents the public and need not be an RN. All the Directors who serve on the AHNCC have been chosen for their skill in and knowledge of holistic nursing and of the process of certification. There is a public member who is not a registered nurse.

The AHNCC is an autonomous body with administrative independence in matters pertaining to specialty certification. The AHNCC maintains a collaborative relationship with but is not involved with the AHNA continuing education, endorsement, or accreditation activities.

The AHNCC defines certification as a qualifying process attesting that an individual, who is already practicing as a registered nurse and demonstrating basic nursing competencies, has met predetermined criteria for basic or advanced specialized practice. In relation to holistic nursing certification, the nurse must demonstrate competencies of specialized nursing practice encompassing holism.

The purpose of a certification process is to provide nurses with a standard they can be measured against, and to be able to declare to the community at large that certain individuals are competent to practice holistic nursing.

AHNCC National Board Certification in holistic nursing is available at the basic (HN-BC) level, which requires a baccalaureate degree, and advanced (AHN-BC) level, which requires a graduate degree. The process for basic certification includes a formal qualitative review of an applicant's portfolio documenting the practice of holistic nursing (RN licensure, academic credentials, holistic nursing experience, continuing education, or successful completion of the certificate program in holistic nursing), and a quantitative certification exam that was developed jointly by the AHNA and the National League of Nursing testing office. The Advanced Certification Exam was developed jointly by the AHNCC and the Professional Testing Service and first offered in March 2005. The process for advanced level certification also requires a qualitative assessment and a quantitative advanced certification exam. Recertification for both basic and advanced levels is completed by documentation of contact hours in holistic nursing.

Further, the AHNCC provides endorsement for university-based undergraduate and graduate nursing programs whose curricula meet the holistic nursing standards in this book (*Holistic Nursing: Scope and Standards of Practice*) so their graduates may sit for the certification exam without providing a qualitative assessment.

Continued Commitment to the Profession

The specialty practice of holistic nursing is generally not well understood. Therefore each holistic nurse must educate other nurses, healthcare providers, professionals, and the public about the role, value, and benefits of holistic nursing, whether it be in direct practice, education, management, or research. Holistic nurses articulate the ideas of the holistic paradigm and the philosophy of the caring–healing model. Jean Watson reminds us that society and the public are searching for something deeper in terms of realizing self-care, self-knowledge, and self-healing potentials. Nurses need to acknowledge the human aspects of practice, attending to people and their experience rather than just focusing on the medical orientation and disease. She concludes that "nurses have a covenant with the public to sustain caring. It is our collective responsibility to transform caring practices into the framework that identifies and gives distinction to nursing as a profession" (Watson 2005, p. 12).

Holistic nurses are committed to continuous, lifelong learning and personal growth for self and others. As role models, they engage in self-assessment and commit to practicing self-care to enhance their physical, psychological, intellectual, social, and spiritual well-being.

Holistic nurses promote the advancement of the profession and holistic nursing by participating in professional and community organizations, writing, publishing, and speaking to professional and lay or public audiences. By engaging in local, state, national, and international forums, they strive to increase the awareness of holistic health issues and the development of holistic care models.

Holistic nurses are particularly attentive to their role as advocates for both people and the environment. They seek to understand the political, social, ethnic, organizational, financial, and discriminatory barriers to holistic care for individuals, population groups, and communities. Holistic nurses work to eliminate these barriers, particularly for the repressed and underserved. They respect and honor people's dignity and freedom to choose among existing alternatives. Holistic nurses assist and empower people to develop self-advocacy skills and make educated life choices. Holistic nurses engage in activities that respect, nurture, and enhance the integral relationship with the earth, contributing to creating an ecosystem the supports the well-being of all life. Acting as teachers, leaders, collaborators, and consultants, they evaluate global health issues and environmental safety, and assist in reducing or eliminating the effects of environmental hazards on the health or welfare of individuals, groups, and communities.

Care of Older Adults

Holistic nursing care is provided to people of all ages across the continuum of care from health promotion and wellness care to acute illness care. Holistic nursing recognizes that older adults represent the predominant population in the healthcare delivery system, a unique population who can benefit greatly from holistic nursing services. Currently, there are more than 36 million people ages 65 or older in the U.S., and this number will increase dramatically by 2011 when many of the baby boomers turn 65. Aging is a multidimensional experience that encompasses the interrelatedness of the body-mind-emotion-spirit-environment. It includes physical, sensory, affective, cognitive, behavioral, sociocultural, and spiritual elements. As aging is a holistic experience, the elderly must be approached in an individualized and comprehensive manner.

As a result of advances in health care during the past century, nurses are caring less frequently for people dying from infections and accidents, major sources of mortality at the turn of the century. Today nurses are often caring for older adults with chronic illnesses, which are a significant source of morbidity and mortality. Older adults dying of infectious processes tend to do so as a result of complications of a chronic illness or debilitation. These chronic conditions contribute significantly to increased healthcare costs. Most of these leading causes of disability and death in the United States are modifiable, and in some cases are preventable. In addition, despite an increased incidence of disease and disability, poor health is not an inevitable consequence of aging.

Adopting healthy lifestyles—getting regular physical exercise, having social support, maintaining a healthy diet, avoiding tobacco and substance use, and receiving regular health-care screenings (e.g., for breast, cervical, and colorectal cancers, for diabetes, and for depression)—can dramatically reduce a person's risk of chronic illnesses.

Not only do a majority of elders experience a chronic condition, but most also have to live with and manage several chronic conditions concurrently. Adopting better lifestyle habits, in conjunction with many of the complementary modalities available to older adults, offers tremendous potential in improving quality of life for older adults, as well as decreasing co-morbidities (e.g., immobility, pain, dementia) associated with chronic illnesses. Many chronic conditions could be aided by a holistic approach and a variety of CAM therapies.

The 1999 National Health Interview Study (U.S. DHHS 1999b) indicated that CAM use increases with age (39% for age 50-plus and 70% for age 85 years and older). Older adults use CAM therapies to treat these common problems:

- Back pain or problems

- Neck pain or problems

- Joint pain or stiffness

- Anxiety

- Depression

Most users of CAM therapies do so without the knowledge or guidance of any healthcare professional. This certainly can pose a risk in geriatric care in that older adults may be:

- Self-diagnosing and self-treating with CAM products and therapies that could delay the diagnosis and perhaps more appropriate treatment for a health condition

- Unknowingly subjecting themselves to complications associated with interactions or adverse reactions to CAM therapies

- Wasting limited funds on CAM products and services that are ineffective for their specific conditions

Nurses can make a critical difference in assuring that older adults receive maximum benefit at minimum risk as they integrate CAM and conventional therapies.

Elders benefit by using holistic CAM therapies because:

- Holistic therapies build on the body's capabilities and are aimed toward strengthening the body's own defenses and healing abilities so that it can do for itself. Strengthened and healthy defenses offer elders benefits that exceed symptom management.

- Total health state is considered and a balanced lifestyle is promoted to control existing health problems, prevent new problems, and enhance general health state.

- Holistic therapies view the person holistically, realizing that people are complex combinations of unique bodies, minds, emotion, and spirits. CAM considers this interconnectedness as it assesses and addresses the physical, mental, emotional, environmental, and spiritual aspects of the person.

- Healing practices are tailored to the individual. This is especially true for older adults, each of whom is the product of an individualized aging process. Whole-person practices offer customized healing measures.

- Holistic therapies empower older adults and encourage self-care. People are taught about self-care practices, guided in using them, and assisted in exploring possible obstacles. Older adults are empowered when they are encouraged to take maximum responsibility for their care. Also, family members and caregivers can be taught simple holistic techniques to use with their loved ones and themselves, thereby empowering the caregivers/family to participate in the elder's care and reduce their own stress.

- The elder is honored by receiving the attention needed. The abbreviated office visit, common in conventional practice, causes many elders to feel that they must be selective in what they share with their healthcare provider. As a result, questions, emotional problems, socioeconomic concerns, and spiritual issues that affect health may not be shared. In contrast, holistic practitioners are more likely to spend time learning about the total person and address needs holistically.

- Most holistic therapies are safer and gentler than conventional therapies. A variety of age-related changes, combined with the high volume and nature of medications used, cause drugs to carry many risks for elders. Although there are conditions for which drugs provide remarkable benefit, there are other conditions that can be managed and improved through lower-risk CAM approaches.

(Adapted from Eliopoulos 2005 and Shelky 2005.)

With the many benefits that can be derived from using CAM and a holistic approach, holistic nurses can best assist elders by helping them to integrate CAM with conventional therapies. This requires that nurses understand the intended and safe use of various CAM therapies, educate elders in appropriate CAM use, and prepare themselves to offer selected CAM therapies as part of their practice.

As part of its continued commitment to improve the quality of health care for older adults and advanced geriatric competence in holistic nursing practice, the AHNA offers a series of continuing education modules on topics related to Geriatric Nursing. These modules were developed through a grant (Nurse Competency in Aging Grant) from the ANA and the John A. Hartford Foundation Institute for Geriatric Nursing, New York University.

AHNA is disseminating the message that competency in geriatric care is relevant for all nurses as the demographics of the population rapidly shift. The AHNA is dedicated to making geriatric care an integral part of holistic nursing education. Additionally, AHNA has launched a geriatric nursing resource on its website for information about caring for older adults as part of holistic nursing practice (www.ahna.org/new/GeroFocus.html).

Current Trends and Issues

(The material in this section has been adapted with permission of Springer Publications from Mariano 2003.)

Trends in Holistic Nursing

The American public is increasingly demanding health care that is compassionate, respectful, provides options, is economically feasible, and is grounded in holistic ideals. A shift is occurring in health care where people desire to be more actively involved in health decision-making. They have expressed their dissatisfaction with conventional (Western) medicine and are calling for a care system that encompasses health, quality of life, and relationship with their providers (Barnes et al. 2004). The American public has pursued alternative and complementary care at an ever-increasing rate. In 1993 David Eisenberg and colleagues published a now-classic study that indicated that one-third (61 million) of Americans were using some form of alternative or complementary form of medicine (Eisenberg et al. 1993). Their continued study on use of complementary/alternative care in 1998 indicated that the use of such modalities not only continued, but sharply increased to 42% (83 million Americans). The total number of visits to providers of complementary care increased by 47%, from 427 million in 1990 to 629 million in 1997 (Eisenberg et al. 1998).

The out-of-pocket dollars spent on complementary/alternative modalities by the American public was $12.2 billion, which exceeded the out-of-pocket expenditures for all U.S. hospitalizations and compared with total out-of-pocket expense for all physician services. The most recent surveys (Barnes et al. 2004 and IOM 2005) indicate that 62% of the American public used some form of complementary/alternative modalities during the previous 12 months and estimate that between $36 to $47 billion was spent on CAM therapies.

A July 2006 survey by Health Forum, a subsidiary of the American Hospital Association (AHA), indicated that 27% of surveyed hospitals (N=1,400) are offering CAM programs to their patients. The reasons cited for offering CAM services are patient demand, clinical effectiveness, desire to treat the "whole person—body, mind, and spirit," attracting new patients, and providing additional services to existing patients.

Western medicine is proving wholly or partially ineffective for a significant proportion of common chronic diseases. Furthermore, highly technological healthcare is too expensive to be universally affordable. Holistic care that promotes health is more cost-effective and culturally acceptable to diverse and disparate populations whose belief systems are more congruent with whole-system and holistic approaches to treatment. The use of alternative methods for economic and cultural reasons by such populations often outweighs their use of conventional treatments.

An issue of CDC's *Advance Data from Vital and Health Statistics* on CAM use in the United States (Barnes et al. 2004) noted characteristics commonly associated with CAM therapies: "Individualized diagnosis and treatment of patients; an emphasis on maximizing the body's inherent healing ability; and treatment of the 'whole' person by addressing their physical, mental, and spiritual attributes rather than focusing on a specific pathogenic process as emphasized in conventional medicine" (p. 2). The National Center for Complementary and Alternative Medicine *Strategic Plan for 2005–2009* (NCCAM 2005) and *Healthy People 2010 Midcourse Review* (U.S. DHHS 2005) have set as priorities enhancing physical and mental health and wellness, preventing disease, and empowering the public to take responsibility for their health.

The White House Commission on CAM Policy (WHCCAMP) *Final Report* (2002) stated that people have come to recognize that a healthy lifestyle can promote wellness and prevent illness and disease, and many individuals have used CAM modalities to attain this goal. Wellness incorporates a broad array of activities and interventions that focus on the physical, mental, spiritual, and emotional aspects of one's life. The effectiveness of the healthcare delivery system in the future will depend on its ability to use all approaches and modalities to contribute to a sound base for promoting health. Early interventions that promote the development of good health habits and attitudes could help modify many of the negative behaviors and lifestyle choices that began in adolescence and continue into old age. The report recommends that:

- more evidence-based teaching about CAM approaches is included in the conventional health professional schools;

- emphasis on the importance of approaches to prevent disease and promote wellness for long-term health of the American people;

- the teaching of the principles and practices of self-care and lifestyle counseling in professional schools be increased in importance, so that health professionals can, in turn, provide this guidance to their patients as well as to improve practitioners' health;

- those in the greatest need, including the chronically ill and those with limited incomes, must have available the most accurate, up-to-date information about which therapies and products may help and which may harm; and

- the education and training of all practitioners should be designed to increase the availability of practitioners knowledgeable in both CAM and conventional practices.

Weeks (2001) outlined several trends in holistic therapies that demonstrate how consumer use is influencing insurance coverage, education, and practice:

- The majority of physicians support the use of at least one or more CAM therapies.

- Approximately two-thirds of health maintenance organizations offered some coverage for CAM services, and that trend is increasing.

- The American Hospital Association has developed a program to educate member institutions on how to offer CAM services.

- Agencies such as Agency for Health Research and Quality, Bureau of Primary Health Care, Center for Disease Control and Prevention

(CDC), Health Care Financing Administration (HCFA), and the Veterans Administration have explored CAM's role in their service delivery systems.

- Integrative clinics that include both CAM and conventional providers are increasing across the country.

This driving force will propel mainstream health care increasingly in this direction, and holistic nurses are in a prime position to meet this need and provide leadership in this national trend.

In the last five to seven years, many conventional healthcare institutions have developed programs, including stress management, energy therapies, healers in the operating rooms, and acupuncture. Programs such as Reiki or Therapeutic Touch for chronic pain, support groups using imagery for breast cancer, and groups espousing meditation for health and wellness are commonly advertised across the United States. Similarly, local pharmacies and health food stores are selling an array of supplements, herbs, homeopathic preparations, vitamins, hormones, and various combinations of these that were not considered marketable five years ago. The number of books, journals, and Web sites devoted to complementary, integrative, and holistic healing practices has also dramatically increased.

Having healthcare providers who have knowledge and skill in promotion of healthful living and integration of complementary/alternative modalities is a critical need for Americans (IOM 2005). Holistic nurses are professionals who have knowledge of a wide range of complementary/alternative/integrative modalities; health promotion/restoration and disease prevention strategies; and relationship-centered, caring ways of healing.

Issues in Holistic Nursing

A number of issues exist or will emerge in holistic nursing's future. Acceptance of holistic nursing's legitimacy, both within nursing as well as other disciplines, is one of the most pressing issues today. Other issues can be categorized into education, research, clinical practice, and policy. It is important to note that because many of these issues face not only holistic nursing but other disciplines as well, an interdisciplinary approach is imperative for success in achieving the desired outcomes.

Education

There are several areas of educational challenge in the holistic arena. With increased use of complementary and alternative therapies by the American public, both students and faculty need knowledge and skill in their use. Of priority is the integration of holistic relationship-centered philosophies and complementary and alternative modalities into nursing curricula. Core content appropriate for both basic and advanced practice programs needs to be identified, and models for integration of both content and practice experiences into existing curricula are necessary. An elective course is not sufficient to imbue this knowledge to future practitioners of nursing. Holistic nurses will need to work with the accrediting bodies of degree programs to ensure that this content is included in educational programs. There is a definitive need for increased scholarship and financial aid to support training in this area. Faculty development programs also will be necessary to support faculty in understanding and integrating holistic philosophy and practices throughout the curriculum.

Licensure and credentialing provide another challenge for holistic nursing. As complementary/alternative medicine has gained national recognition, state boards of nursing began to attend to the regulation issues. In 2001, Captain Andrew Sparber of the U.S. Public Health Service conducted a study to ascertain the number of boards of nursing that had a formal policy, position, or inclusion of complementary therapies under the scope of practice (Sparber 2001). He found that 25 states (47%) had statements or positions that included specific complementary therapies or examples of these practices, 7 (13%) were discussing the topic, and 21 (40%) had not formally addressed the topic but did not discourage these practices. It will be important in the future to monitor state boards of nursing for evidence of their recognition and support of integrative nursing practice and requirements that include CAM for nursing educational program approval. Finally, holistic nursing has the challenge of working with the state boards to incorporate this content into the National Council Licensure Examination, thus ensuring the credibility of this practice knowledge.

To improve the competency of practitioners and the quality of services, CAM education and training needs to continue beyond basic and advanced academic education. Continuing education programs at national and regional specialty organizations' meetings and conferences may assist in meeting this need. Working with practitioners in other areas of nursing to increase their understanding of the philosophical and theoretical foundations of holistic nursing practices (e.g., intention, presence, and centering) will also be a role of holistic nurses.

Research

Research in the area of holistic nursing will become increasingly important in the future. There is a great need for an evidence base establishing the effectiveness and efficacy of complementary/alternative therapies. However, one of the formidable tasks for nurses will be to identify and describe outcomes of CAM therapies such as healing, well-being, and harmony in order to develop instruments to measure these outcomes. Presently, most outcome measures are based on physical or disease symptomatology. In addition, methodologies need to be expanded to capture the wholeness of the individual's experience, because the philosophy of the CAM therapies rests on a paradigm of wholeness.

Nurses need to address how to secure funding for their holistic research. They need to apply to National Institutes of Health (NIH) centers and Institutes other than just the National Institute of Nursing Research for funding, particularly the National Center for Complementary and Alternative Medicine. But hand in hand with this is the need for nurses to be represented on study sections and review panels to educate and convince the biomedical/NIH community about the value of nursing research; the need for models of research focusing on health promotion and disease prevention, wellness, and self-care instead of just the disease model; and the importance of a variety of designs and research methodologies including qualitative studies, rather than sole reliance on randomized controlled trials.

An area of responsibility for advanced practice holistic nurses is the dissemination of their research findings to various media sources (e.g., television, newsprint) and at non-nursing, interdisciplinary conferences. Publishing in non-nursing journals and serving on editorial boards of non-nursing journals also broadens the appreciation of other disciplines for nursing's role in setting the agenda and conducting research in the area of holism and CAM.

Clinical Practice

Clinical care models reflecting holistic assessment, treatment, health, healing, and caring are important in the development of holistic practice and CAM integration. Implementing holistic and humanistic models in today's healthcare environment will require a paradigm shift for the many providers who subscribe to a disease model of care. Such an acceptance poses an enormous challenge. Holistic nurses with their education and experience are the logical leaders in integrative care and must advance that position.

Addressing the nursing shortage in this country is crucial to the health of our nation. Nurses often leave the profession or frequently change jobs because of unhumanistic and chaotic work environments and professional and personal burnout. Holistic nurses, through their knowledge of caring cultures and stress management techniques, have an extraordinary opportunity to influence and improve the healthcare environments, both for healthcare providers and clients/patients.

Policy

Three major policy issues face holistic nursing in the future: reimbursement, regulation, and access. Public or private policies regarding coverage of and reimbursement for healthcare services play a crucial role in shaping the healthcare system and will play a crucial role in deciding the future of wellness, health promotion, and CAM in the nation's healthcare system. Often CAM is offered as a supplemental benefit rather than as a core or basic benefit, and many third-party payers do not cover such services at all. Coverage of and reimbursement for most services depend on the provider's ability to legally furnish services within the scope of practice. The legal authority to practice is given by the state in which services are provided.

Reimbursement of advanced practice nurses also depends on appropriate credentialing. Holistic nurses will need to work with Medicare and other third-party payers, insurance groups, boards of nursing, healthcare policy makers, legislators, and other professional nursing organizations to ensure that holistic nurses are appropriately reimbursed for services rendered. Another issue regarding reimbursement is the fact that the effectiveness of CAM is influenced by the holistic focus and integrative skill of the provider. Consequently, reimbursement must be included for the process of holistic/integrative care, not just for providing a specific modality.

There are many barriers to the use of holistic therapies by the increasing number of users, providing yet another challenge for holistic nurses.

Barriers include lack of awareness of the therapies and their benefits, uncertainty about their effectiveness, inability to pay for them, and limited availability of qualified providers. Access is even more difficult for rural populations; uninsured or underinsured populations; special populations, such as racial and ethnic minorities; and vulnerable populations, such as the elderly and the chronically and terminally ill (WHCCAMP 2002). Holistic nurses have a responsibility to educate the public more fully about health promotion and complementary/alternative modalities and qualified practitioners and to assist people to make informed choices among the array of healthcare alternatives and individual providers. Holistic nurses also must actively participate in the political arena as leaders in this movement to ensure quality, an increased focus on wellness, and access and affordability for all.

Holistic nurses, by developing theoretical and empirical knowledge and caring/healing approaches, will advance holistic nursing practice and education and contribute significantly to the formalization and credibility of this work. They will provide the leadership in the profession in research, the development of educational models, and the integration of a more holistic approach in nursing practice and health care.

Standards of Holistic Nursing Practice

Overarching Philosophical Principles of Holistic Nursing

Holistic nurses express, contribute to, and promote an understanding of the following: a philosophy of nursing that values healing as the desired outcome; the human health experience as a complex, dynamic relationship of health, illness, disease, and wellness; the scientific foundations of nursing practice; and nursing as an art. It is based on the following overarching philosophical tenets that are embedded in every standard of practice.

Principles of Holistic Nursing

The following principles underlie holistic nursing:

Person

- There is unity, totality, and connectedness of everyone and every-thing (body, mind, emotion, spirit, sexuality, age, environment, social/cultural, belief systems, relationships, context).

- Human beings are unique and inherently good.

- People are able to find meaning and purpose in their own life, experiences, and illness.

- All people have an innate power and capacity for self-healing. Health/illness is subjectively described and determined by the view of the individual. Therefore, the person is honored in all phases of his/her healing process regardless of expectations or outcomes.

- People/persons/individuals identify (are) the recipient(s) of holistic nursing services. These can be clients, patients, families, significant others, populations, or communities. They may be ill and within the healthcare delivery system or well, moving toward personal better-ment to enhance well-being.

Healing/Health

- Health and illness are natural and a part of life, learning, and movement toward change and development.

- Health is seen as balance, integration, harmony, right relationship, and the betterment of well-being, not just the absence of disease. Healing can take place without cure. The focus is on health promotion/disease prevention/health restoration/lifestyle patterns and habits, as well as symptom relief.

- Illness is considered a teacher and an opportunity for self-awareness and growth as part of the life process. Symptoms are respected as messages.

- People as active partners in the healing process are empowered when they take some control of their own lives, health, and well-being, including personal choices and relationships.

- Treatment is a process that considers the root of the problem, not merely treating the obvious signs and symptoms.

Practice

- Practice is a science (critical thinking, reflection, evidence/research/ theory as underlying practice) and an art (intuition, creativity, presence, and self/personal knowing as integral to practice).

- The values and ethic of holism, caring, moral insight, dignity, integrity, competence, responsibility, accountability, and legality underlie holistic nursing practice.

- There are various philosophies and paradigms of health, illness, healing, and approaches/models for the delivery of health care, both in the United States and in other cultures, that need to be understood and utilized.

- Older adults represent the predominant population served by nurses.

- Public policy and the healthcare delivery system influence the health and well-being of society and professional nursing.

Nursing Roles

- The nurse is part of the healing environment using warmth, compassion, caring, authenticity, respect, trust, and relationship as instruments of healing in and of themselves.

- Using conventional nursing interventions as well as holistic/ complementary/alternative/integrative modalities that enhance the body-mind-emotion-spirit-environment connectedness to foster healing, health, wholenesss, and well-being of people.

- Collaborating and partnering with all constituencies in the health process including the person receiving care and family, community, peers, and other disciplines. Using principles and skills of cooperation, alliance, and respect, and honoring the contributions of all.

- Participating in the change process to develop more caring cultures in which to practice and learn.

- Assisting nurses to nurture and heal themselves.

- Participating in activities that contribute to the improvement of communities and the environment and to the betterment of public health.

- Acting as an advocate for the rights of and equitable distribution and access to health care for all persons, especially vulnerable populations.

- Honoring the ecosystem and our relationship with and need to preserve it, as we are all connected.

Self-Care

- The nurse's self-reflection and self-assessment, self-care, healing, and personal development are necessary for service to others and growth/change in one's own well-being and understanding of one's own personal journey.

- The nurse values oneself and one's calling to holistic nursing as a life purpose.

Holistic nursing practice is guided by the holistic caring process, whether used with individuals, families, population groups, or communities. This process involves assessment, diagnosis, outcome identification, planning, implementation, and evaluation. It encompasses all significant actions taken in providing culturally, ethically, respectful, compassionate, and relevant holistic nursing care to all persons.

STANDARDS OF PRACTICE

STANDARD 1. ASSESSMENT
The holistic nurse collects comprehensive data pertinent to the person's health or situation.

Measurement Criteria:

The holistic registered nurse:

- Collects comprehensive data including but not limited to physical, functional, psychosocial, emotional, mental, sexual, cultural, age-related, environmental, spiritual/transpersonal, and energy field assessments in a systematic and ongoing process while honoring the uniqueness of the person.

- Identifies areas such as the person's health and cultural practices, values, beliefs, preferences, meanings of health/illness, lifestyle patterns, family issues, and risk behaviors and context.

- Involves the person, family, significant others, caregivers, other healthcare providers, and environment as appropriate in holistic data collection.

- Prioritizes data collection activities based on the person's immediate condition or anticipated needs of the person or situation.

- Uses appropriate evidence-based assessment techniques and instruments in collecting pertinent data as a basis for holistic care.

- Uses analytical models and problem-solving tools.

- Synthesizes available data, information, and knowledge relevant to the situation to identify patterns and variances as they relate to the whole person within the life context.

- Documents and stores relevant data in a retrievable format that is secure and confidential.

- Incorporates various types of knowing, including intuition, when gathering data from the person and validates this intuitive knowledge with the person when appropriate.

Continued ▶

Additional Measurement Criteria for the Holistic Advanced Practice Registered Nurse:

The holistic advanced practice registered nurse:

- Initiates and interprets diagnostic procedures relevant to the person's current status.

- Recognizes the person as the authority on his/her own health experience.

- Elicits and uses client narratives to reveal the context and complexity of the health experience.

- Explores the meanings of the symbolic language expressing itself in areas such as dreams, images, symbols, sensations, and prayers that are a part of the individual's health experience.

STANDARD 2. DIAGNOSIS OR HEALTH ISSUES
The holistic nurse analyzes the assessment data to determine the diagnosis or health issues expressed as actual or potential patterns/problems/needs that are related to health, wellness, disease, or illness.

Measurement Criteria:

The holistic registered nurse:

- Derives the diagnosis or health issues based on holistic assessment data.

- Assists the person to explore the meaning of the health/disease experience.

- Validates the diagnosis or health issues with the person, family/ significant other, and other healthcare providers when possible and appropriate.

- Documents diagnoses or health issues in a manner that facilitates the determination of the expected outcomes and plan.

Additional Measurement Criteria for the Holistic Advanced Practice Registered Nurse:

The holistic advanced practice registered nurse:

- Systematically compares and contrasts clinical findings with normal and abnormal variations and development events in formulating a differential diagnosis.

- Utilizes complex data and information obtained during interview, examination, and diagnostic procedures in determining diagnosis.

- Establishes the diagnoses reflecting the level of acuity, severity, and complexity of health patterns/challenges/needs.

- Assists staff in developing and maintaining competency in the diagnostic process.

Standard 3: Outcomes Identification
The holistic registered nurse identifies outcomes for a plan individualized to the person or the situation.

The holistic nurse values the evolution and the process of healing as it unfolds. This implies that specific unfolding outcomes may not be evident immediately due to the non-linear nature of the healing process so that both expected/anticipated and evolving outcomes are considered.

Measurement Criteria:

The holistic registered nurse:

- Involves the person, family, significant others, and other healthcare providers in formulating outcomes when possible and appropriate.

- Derives culturally appropriate outcomes from the diagnoses.

- Considers associated risks, benefits, costs, current scientific evidence, and clinical expertise when formulating outcomes.

- Defines outcomes in terms of the person; the individual's values and beliefs, preferences, age, spiritual practices; ethical considerations, environment, or situation, considering associated risks, benefits, costs, and current scientific evidence.

- Partners with the person to identify realistic goals based on the person's present and potential capabilities and quality of life.

- Assists the person to understand the potential for unfolding outcomes due to the nature of healing.

- Includes a realistic time estimate for attainment of outcomes.

- Develops outcomes that provide direction for continuity of care.

- Modifies outcomes based on changes in the status or preference of the person or evaluation of the situation.

- Documents outcomes as measurable goals.

- Focuses on the person's attaining, maintaining, or regaining health, healing, well-being, or peaceful dying while honoring all phases of her/his healing process regardless of expectations or outcomes.

Additional Measurement Criteria for the Holistic Advanced Practice Registered Nurse:

The holistic advanced practice registered nurse:

- Identifies outcomes that incorporate scientific evidence and are achievable through implementation of evidence-based practices.

- Identifies outcomes that incorporate patient satisfaction, the person's understanding and meanings in their unique patterns and processes, quality of life, cost and clinical effectiveness, and continuity and consistency among providers.

- Supports the use of clinical guidelines for positive outcomes related to the person's healing.

STANDARD 4. PLANNING
The holistic registered nurse develops a plan that identifies strategies and alternatives to attain outcomes.

Measurement Criteria:

The holistic registered nurse:

- Develops in partnership with the person an individualized plan considering the person's characteristics or situation including, but not limited to, values, beliefs, spiritual and health practices, preferences, choices, age and cultural appropriateness, environmental sensitivity.

- Develops the plan in conjunction with the person, family, and others, as appropriate.

- Includes strategies within the plan that address each of the identified diagnoses, health issues, or opportunities that may include strategies for promotion and restoration of health and well-being; prevention of illness, injury, and disease; or peaceful dying.

- Collaborates and participates in interdisciplinary/multidisciplinary teams to provide for continuity within the plan.

- Incorporates an implementation pathway or time line within the plan.

- Establishes the plan priorities with the person, family, and others, as appropriate.

- Utilizes the plan to provide direction to other members of the healthcare team.

- Defines the plan to reflect current statutes, rules and regulations, and standards.

- Integrates current trends, research, and evidence-based interventions affecting care in the planning process.

- Considers the economic impact of the plan.

- Includes strategies for health, wholeness, and growth from infant to elder.

- Establishes practice settings and safe space and time for both the nurse and person/family/significant others to explore suggested, potential, and alternative options.

- Uses standardized language or recognized terminology to document the plan.

Additional Measurement Criteria for the Holistic Advanced Practice Registered Nurse:

The holistic advanced practice registered nurse:

- Identifies assessment, diagnostic strategies, and therapeutic interventions within the plan and therapeutic effects and side effects that reflect current evidence, including data, research, literature, and expert clinical knowledge and the person's experiences.

- Selects or designs, in partnership with the person, strategies to meet the multifaceted holistic needs of complex individuals.

- Includes the synthesis of the person's values, beliefs, preferences, and choices regarding nursing and medical therapies within the plan.

- Uses linguistic and symbolic language including but not limited to word associations, dreams, storytelling, and journals to explore with individuals the possibilities and options.

STANDARD 5. IMPLEMENTATION
The holistic registered nurse implements the identified plan in partnership with the person.

Measurement Criteria:

The holistic registered nurse:

- Partners with the person/family/significant others/caregiver to implement the plan in a safe and timely manner.

- Documents the implementation and any modifications, including changes to or omissions from the identified plan.

- Utilizes evidence-based interventions and treatments specific to the diagnosis or problem.

- Utilizes community resources and systems to implement the plan.

- Collaborates with nursing colleagues and others to implement the plan.

- Promotes the person's capacity for the highest level of participation and problem solving, honoring the person's choices and unique healing journey.

Additional Measurement Criteria for the Holistic Advanced Practice Registered Nurse:

The holistic advanced practice registered nurse:

- Facilitates utilization of systems and community resources to implement the plan.

- Supports collaboration with nursing colleagues and other disciplines to implement the plan for individuals, families, groups, and communities that integrates biomedical, complementary, and alternative approaches to healing.

- Incorporates new knowledge and strategies to initiate change in nursing care practices if desired outcomes are not achieved.

STANDARD 5A: COORDINATION OF CARE
The holistic registered nurse coordinates care delivery.

Measurement Criteria:

The holistic registered nurse:

- Coordinates implementation of the plan.

- Documents the coordination of the care.

- Assists the person to recognize alternatives by identifying options for care choices.

Additional Measurement Criteria for the Holistic Advanced Practice Registered Nurse:

The holistic advanced practice registered nurse:

- Provides leadership in the coordination of multidisciplinary health care for integrated delivery of person care services.

- Synthesizes data and information to prescribe necessary system and community support measures, including environmental modifications.

- Coordinates system, environmental, human, and community resources that enhance delivery of care across continuums and over time.

STANDARD 5B: HEALTH TEACHING AND HEALTH PROMOTION
The holistic registered nurse employs strategies to promote holistic health/wellness and a safe environment.

Measurement Criteria:

The holistic registered nurse:

- Provides health teaching to individuals, families, and significant others or caregivers that enhances the body-mind-emotion-spirit-environment connection by addressing such topics as:

  - Healthy lifestyles

  - Risk-reducing behaviors

  - Developmental need

  - Activities of daily living

  - Preventive self-care

  - Living with changes secondary to illness and treatment

  - Stress management

  - Opportunities to enhance well-being

- Uses health promotion and health teaching methods appropriate to the situation and the individual's values, beliefs, health practices, age, learning needs, readiness and ability to learn, language preference, spirituality, culture, and socioeconomic status.

- Seeks ongoing opportunities for feedback and evaluation of the effectiveness of the strategies used.

- Educates others by demonstrating a holistic philosophy and ethic that value all ways of knowing and learning.

- Provides appropriate information including but not limited to intended effects and potential adverse effects of the proposed prescribed agents/treatments, costs, complementary/alternative/holistic treatments and procedures, and the effects of single and multiple interventions on the person's health and functioning.

- Assists others to access their own inner wisdom that may provide opportunities to enhance and support growth, development, and wholeness.

Additional Measurement Criteria for the Holistic Advanced Practice Registered Nurse:

The holistic advanced practice registered nurse:

- Synthesizes empirical evidence on risk behaviors, decision-making about life choices, learning theories, behavioral change theories, motivational theories, epidemiology, and other related theories and frameworks when designing holistic health information and education.

- Designs health information and education appropriate to the individual's developmental level, learning needs, readiness to learn, and cultural values and beliefs.

- Evaluates health information resources, such as the Internet, within the area of practice for accuracy, readability, and comprehensibility to help the person access quality health information.

- Creates educational environments that are safe for the exploration necessary for learning.

Standard 5c: Consultation
The holistic advanced practice registered nurse provides consultation to influence the identified plan, enhance the abilities of others, and effect change.

Measurement Criteria for the Holistic Advanced Practice Registered Nurse:

The holistic advanced practice registered nurse:

- Synthesizes clinical data, theoretical frameworks, organizational structures, belief/value systems, and evidence when providing consultation.

- Facilitates the effectiveness of a consultation by involving all stakeholders including the individual in decision-making and negotiating role responsibilities.

- Communicates consultation recommendations that facilitate change.

STANDARD 5D: PRESCRIPTIVE AUTHORITY AND TREATMENT

The holistic advanced practice registered nurse uses prescriptive authority, procedures, referrals, treatments, and therapies in accordance with state and federal laws and regulations.

Measurement Criteria for the Holistic Advanced Practice Registered Nurse:

The holistic advanced practice registered nurse:

- Prescribes treatments, therapies, and procedures based on evidence, research, current knowledge, and practice considering the person's holistic healthcare needs and choices.

- Prescribes pharmacologic agents based on a current knowledge of pharmacology and physiology.

- Uses advanced knowledge of pharmacology, psychoneuroimmunology, nutritional supplements, herbal and homeopathic remedies, and a variety of complementary and alternative therapies in prescribing.

- Prescribes specific pharmacologic agents and/or treatments based on: clinical indicators; the person's status, needs, and age; the results of diagnostic and laboratory tests; and the person's beliefs, values, and choices.

- Prescribes holistic therapies that enhance body-mind-emotion-spirit-environment connectedness and foster healing and wholeness.

- Evaluates therapeutic and potential adverse effects of pharmacological and non-pharmacological treatments including but not limited to drug/herbal/homeopathic regimens as well as drug/herbal/homeopathic side effects and interactions.

- Provides individuals with information about intended effects and potential adverse effects of proposed prescriptive therapies.

- Analyzes the effects of single and multiple interventions on the person's health and functioning.

- Provides information about costs and alternative treatments and procedures, as appropriate.

STANDARD 6: EVALUATION
The holistic registered nurse evaluates progress toward attainment of outcomes while recognizing and honoring the continuing holistic nature of the healing process.

Measurement Criteria:

The holistic registered nurse:

- Conducts a holistic, systematic, ongoing, and criterion-based evaluation of the outcomes in relation to the structures and processes prescribed by the plan and the indicated time line.

- Collaborates with the person and others involved in the care or situation in the evaluative process.

- Evaluates, in partnership with the person, the effectiveness of the planned strategies in relation to the person's responses and the attainment of the expected and unfolding outcomes.

- Documents the results of the evaluation.

- Uses ongoing assessment data to mutually revise, with the person, family, and health team, the diagnoses, outcomes, plan, and the implementation, as needed.

- Disseminates the results to the person and others involved in the care or situation as appropriate, in accordance with state and federal laws and regulations.

Additional Measurement Criteria for the Holistic Advanced Practice Registered Nurse:

The holistic advanced practice registered nurse:

- Evaluates in partnership with the person the accuracy of the diagnosis and the effectiveness of the interventions in relationship to the person's attainment of expected and evolving outcomes and changes of meaning in the person's health experience.

- Synthesizes the results of the evaluation analyses to determine the impact of the plan on the affected individuals, families, groups, communities, and institutions.

- Uses the results of the evaluation analyses to make or recommend process or structural changes, including policy, procedure, and/or protocol documentation, as appropriate to improve holistic care.

STANDARDS OF PROFESSIONAL PERFORMANCE

STANDARD 7: QUALITY OF PRACTICE
The holistic registered nurse systematically enhances the quality and effectiveness of holistic nursing practice.

Measurement Criteria:

The holistic registered nurse:

- Demonstrates quality by documenting the application of the nursing process in a responsible, accountable, and ethical manner.

- Uses the results of quality improvement activities to initiate changes in holistic nursing practice and in the healthcare delivery system.

- Uses creativity and innovation in holistic nursing practice to improve care delivery.

- Incorporates new knowledge to initiate changes in holistic nursing practice if desired outcomes are not achieved.

- Participates in quality improvement activities for holistic nursing practice. Such activities may include:

  - Identifying aspects of practice important for quality monitoring

  - Using indicators developed to monitor quality and effectiveness of holistic nursing practice

  - Collecting data to monitor quality and effectiveness of holistic nursing practice

  - Analyzing quality data to identify opportunities for improving holistic nursing practice

  - Formulating recommendations to improve holistic nursing practice or outcomes

  - Implementing activities to enhance the quality of holistic nursing practice

  - Developing, implementing, and evaluating policies, procedures, and/or guidelines to improve the quality of practice

Continued ▶

- Participating on interdisciplinary teams to evaluate clinical care or health services
- Participating in efforts to minimize costs and unnecessary duplication
- Analyzing factors related to safety, satisfaction, effectiveness, and cost/benefit options
- Analyzing organizational systems for barriers
- Implementing processes to remove or decrease barriers to holistic care within organizational systems
- Working toward creating organizations that value sacred space and environments that enhance healing

Additional Measurement Criteria for the Holistic Advanced Practice Registered Nurse:

The holistic advanced practice registered nurse:

- Obtains and maintains professional certification in the area of expertise.
- Develops indicators to monitor quality and effectiveness of holistic nursing practice.
- Designs quality improvement initiatives.
- Implements initiatives to evaluate the need for change.
- Evaluates the practice environment and quality of holistic nursing care rendered in relation to existing evidence and feedback from individuals and significant others, identifying opportunities for the generation and use of research.

STANDARD 8: EDUCATION
The holistic registered nurse attains knowledge and competency that reflects current nursing practice.

Measurement Criteria:

The holistic registered nurse:

- Participates in ongoing educational activities related to appropriate knowledge bases for holistic care and professional issues.

- Demonstrates a commitment to lifelong learning through self-reflection and inquiry to identify learning and personal growth needs.

- Seeks experiences that reflect current practice and population/age-related needs in order to maintain skills and competence in clinical practice and dimensions of the holistic nurse role.

- Acquires knowledge and skills appropriate to the holistic nursing specialty area, practice setting, role, or situation.

- Maintains professional records that provide evidence of competency and lifelong learning.

- Seeks experiences and formal and independent learning activities to maintain and develop clinical and professional skills and knowledge and personal growth.

Additional Measurement Criteria for the Holistic Advanced Practice Registered Nurse:

The holistic advanced practice registered nurse:

- Uses current healthcare research findings and other evidence to expand clinical knowledge, enhance role performance, and increase knowledge of professional issues and changes in national standards for practice and trends in holistic care.

STANDARD 9: PROFESSIONAL PRACTICE EVALUATION

The holistic registered nurse evaluates one's own nursing practice in relation to professional practice standards and guidelines, relevant statutes, rules, and regulations.

Measurement Criteria:

The holistic registered nurse's practice reflects the application of knowledge of current practice standards, guidelines, statutes, rules, and regulations.

The holistic registered nurse:

- Reflects on one's practice and how one's own personal, cultural, and/or spiritual beliefs, experiences, biases, education, and values may affect care given to individuals/families/communities.

- Provides age-appropriate care from infant to elder in a culturally and ethnically sensitive manner.

- Engages in self-evaluation of practice on a regular basis, identifying areas of strength as well as areas in which professional development and personal growth would be beneficial.

- Obtains informal feedback regarding one's own holistic practice from individuals receiving care, peers, professional colleagues, and others.

- Participates in systematic peer review as appropriate.

- Takes action to achieve goals identified from evaluation process.

- Provides rationales for practice beliefs, decisions, and actions as part of the informal and formal evaluation processes.

Additional Measurement Criteria for the Holistic Advanced Practice Registered Nurse:

The holistic advanced practice registered nurse:

- Engages in a formal process, seeking feedback regarding one's own practice from individuals receiving care, peers, professional colleagues, and others.

STANDARD 10: COLLEGIALITY
The holistic registered nurse interacts with and contributes to the professional development of peers and colleagues.

Measurement Criteria:

The holistic registered nurse:

- Shares knowledge and skills with peers and colleagues as evidenced by such activities as patient care conferences or presentations at formal or informal meetings.

- Recognizes expertise and competency of diverse disciplines and approaches to health care.

- Provides peers with feedback regarding their practice and/or role performance in a constructive and sincere manner.

- Interacts with peers and colleagues to enhance one's own holistic nursing practice, personal development, and/or role performance.

- Maintains compassionate and caring relationships with peers and colleagues.

- Contributes to an environment that is conducive to enhancing the education of healthcare professionals about holism.

- Promotes work environments conducive to support, understanding, respect, health, healing, caring, wholeness, and harmony.

Additional Measurement Criteria for the Holistic Advanced Practice Registered Nurse:

The holistic advanced practice registered nurse:

- Models expert holistic nursing practice to interdisciplinary team members and healthcare consumers.

- Mentors other registered nurses and colleagues as appropriate.

- Participates with interdisciplinary teams that contribute to role development and advanced holistic nursing practice and holistic health care.

- Establishes practice environments that recognize and value holistic communication as fundamental to holistic care.

Standards of Professional Performance

STANDARD 11: COLLABORATION
The holistic registered nurse collaborates with the person, family, and others in the conduct of holistic nursing practice.

Measurement Criteria:

The holistic registered nurse:

- Communicates with the person, family, significant others, caregivers, and interdisciplinary healthcare providers regarding the person's care and the holistic nurse's role in the provision of that care.

- Collaborates in creating a documented plan, focused on outcomes and decisions related to care and delivery of services, that indicates communication with individuals receiving care, families, and others as appropriate.

- Partners with others to enhance holistic care in order to effect change and generate positive outcomes through knowledge of the person or situation.

- Documents referrals, including provisions for continuity of care.

- Understands, utilizes, and refers to a range of approaches and therapies from diverse disciplines and systems of care as appropriate.

Additional Measurement Criteria for the Holistic Advanced Practice Registered Nurse:

The holistic advanced practice registered nurse:

- Partners with other disciplines to enhance holistic care through interdisciplinary activities such as education, consultation, management, technological development, or research opportunities.

- Facilitates an interdisciplinary process with other members of the healthcare team that enhances the contribution of all.

- Documents plan, communications, rationales for plan changes, and collaborative discussions.

- Facilitates the negotiation of holistic/complementary/alternative/ integrative and conventional healthcare services for continuity of care and program planning.

STANDARD 12: ETHICS
The holistic registered nurse integrates ethical provisions in all areas of practice.

Measurement Criteria:

The holistic registered nurse:

- Uses *Code of Ethics for Nurses with Interpretive Statements* (ANA 2001) and *Position Statement on Holistic Nursing Ethics* (AHNA 2007) to guide practice and articulate the moral foundation of holistic nursing.

- Identifies the ethics of caring and its contribution to unity of self, others, nature, and God/Life Force/Absolute/Transcendent as central to holistic nursing practice.

- Delivers care in a manner that preserves and protects the person's autonomy, dignity, rights, values, and beliefs.

- Protects and maintains the person's personal privacy and confidentiality within legal and regulatory parameters.

- Respects the person's choices and health trajectory, which may be incongruent with conventional wisdom.

- Serves as an advocate in assisting the person in developing skills for self-advocacy and making educated choices about his/her care.

- Maintains a therapeutic and professional person–nurse relationship with appropriate professional role boundaries.

- Engages in self-assessment and demonstrates a commitment to practicing self-care strategies to enhance physical, psychological, intellectual, sociological, and spiritual well-being, manage stress, and connect with self and others.

- Contributes to resolving ethical issues of individuals, colleagues, or systems as evidenced in such activities as participating on ethics committees.

- Reports illegal, incompetent, or impaired practices.

- Recognizes that the well-being of the ecosystem of the planet is a determining condition for the well-being of human beings.

Continued ▶

- Engages in activities that respect, nurture, and enhance the integral relationship with the earth, and advocates for the well-being of the global community's economy, education, and social justice.

- Advocates for the rights of vulnerable, repressed, or underserved populations by such activities as:

  - Acting on behalf of individuals, families, groups, and communities who cannot seek or demand ethical treatment on their own

  - Seeking to eliminate barriers such as affordability and accessibility that create added risks for persons of varied racial, ethnic, and social backgrounds, as well as the elderly and children

  - Advocating for other nurses and colleagues

- Values all life experiences as opportunities to find personal meaning and cultivate self-awareness, self-reflection, and growth.

Additional Measurement Criteria for the Holistic Advanced Practice Registered Nurse:

The holistic advanced practice registered nurse:

- Informs the person of the risks, benefits, and outcomes of health-care regimens.

- Participates in interdisciplinary teams that address ethical risks, benefits, and outcomes.

- Engages others to incorporate a holistic perspective of ethical situations and decision-making.

- Actively contributes to creating an ecosystem that supports well-being for all life.

Standard 13: Research
The holistic registered nurse integrates research into practice.

Measurement Criteria:

The holistic registered nurse:

- Utilizes the best available evidence, including theories and research findings, to guide practice decisions.

- Actively and ethically participates in research activities related to holistic health at various levels appropriate to the holistic nurse's level of education and position. Such activities may include:

  - Identifying problems specific to nursing research (person care and nursing practice)

  - Participating in data collection (surveys, pilot projects, formal studies)

  - Participating in a formal committee or program

  - Sharing research activities and/or findings with individuals/families/peers, those in other disciplines, and others

  - Systematically inquiring into healing, wholeness, cultural, spiritual, and health issues by conducting research or supporting and utilizing the research of others

  - Critically analyzing and interpreting research for application to holistic practice

  - Using research findings in the development of policies, procedures, and standards of practice in holistic person care

  - Incorporating research as a basis for learning

- Contributes to conducting research and applying research findings that link environmental hazards and human response patterns.

Continued ▶

Additional Measurement Criteria for the Holistic Advanced Practice Registered Nurse:

The holistic advanced practice registered nurse:

- Contributes to nursing knowledge by conducting or synthesizing research that discovers, examines, and evaluates knowledge, theories, philosophies, context, criteria, and creative approaches to improve holistic healthcare practice.

- Formally disseminates research findings through activities such as presentations, publications, consultations, and journal clubs for a variety of audiences including nursing, other disciplines, and the public to improve holistic care and further develop the foundation and practice of holistic nursing.

- Creates ways to study the integration of body-mind-emotion-spirit-environment therapies to achieve optimal care outcomes.

- Participates with others to identify research questions or areas for inquiry and set research priorities that have high significance in understanding and/or improving health/wellness promotion and disease prevention; the quality of life; spirituality; cultural beliefs and health practices; and healing and well-being.

STANDARD 14: RESOURCE UTILIZATION
The holistic registered nurse considers factors related to safety, effectiveness, cost, and impact on practice in the planning and delivery of nursing services.

Measurement Criteria:

The holistic registered nurse:

- Evaluates factors such as safety, effectiveness, availability, cost and benefits, efficiencies, and impact on practice when choosing practice options that would result in the same expected outcome.

- Assists the person, family, and significant others or caregivers, as appropriate, in identifying and securing appropriate and available services to address health-related needs.

- Identifies discriminatory healthcare practices as they impact the person and engages in effective nondiscriminatory practices.

- Assigns or delegates tasks based on the needs and condition of the person, potential for harm, stability of the person's condition, complexity of the task, and predictability of the outcome.

- Assists the person, family, and significant others in becoming informed consumers about the health promotion options, costs, risks, and benefits of treatment and care.

Additional Measurement Criteria for the Holistic Advanced Practice Registered Nurse:

The holistic advanced practice registered nurse:

- Utilizes organizational and community resources to formulate multidisciplinary or interdisciplinary plans of care.

- Develops innovative solutions for the person's care needs/challenges/problems that address effective resource utilization and maintenance of quality.

- Develops evaluation strategies to demonstrate cost effectiveness, cost benefit, and efficiency factors associated with holistic nursing practice.

STANDARD 15: LEADERSHIP
The holistic registered nurse provides leadership in the professional practice setting and the profession.

Measurement Criteria:

The holistic registered nurse:

- Engages in teamwork as a team player and a team builder.

- Works to create and maintain healthy work environments conducive to enhancing healing, wholeness, and harmony in local, regional, national, or international communities.

- Displays the ability to define a clear vision, associated goals, and a plan to implement and measure progress toward holistic health care.

- Demonstrates a commitment to continuous, lifelong learning and personal growth for self and others.

- Teaches others to succeed, by mentoring and other strategies.

- Exhibits creativity and flexibility through times of change.

- Demonstrates energy, excitement, and a passion for quality holistic work.

- Willingly accepts mistakes by self and others, thereby creating a culture in which risk-taking is both safe and expected.

- Inspires loyalty through valuing of people as the most precious asset in an organization.

- Directs the coordination of care across settings and among caregivers, including oversight of licensed and unlicensed personnel in any assigned or delegated tasks.

- Serves in key roles in the work setting to advance the philosophy and role of holistic nursing by participating on committees, councils, and administrative teams.

- Promotes advancement of the profession through participation in professional organizations and focusing on strategies that bring unity and healing to the nursing profession.

- Engages in local, state, national, and international levels to expand the knowledge and practice of holistic nursing and awareness of holistic health issues.

Additional Measurement Criteria for the Holistic Advanced Practice Registered Nurse:

The holistic advanced practice registered nurse:

- Works to influence decision-making bodies to improve holistic, integrated care.

- Provides direction to enhance the effectiveness of the healthcare team.

- Initiates and revises protocols or guidelines to reflect evidence-based practice, to reflect accepted changes in care management, or to address emerging problems such as the growing elderly population.

- Promotes communication of information and advancement of the profession and holistic nursing through writing, publishing, and presentations for professional or lay/public audiences.

- Designs innovations to effect change in practice and to improve holistic health outcomes.

- Articulates the ideas underpinning holistic nursing philosophy, placing these ideas in a historical, philosophical, and scientific context while projecting future trends in thinking by such activities as:

  - Applying, teaching, mentoring, and leading others in developing holistic care models and providing holistic integrated care

  - Leading organizations in creating therapeutic environments that value holistic caring, social support, and healing, where individuals feel connected, supported, and valued

  - Understanding the political, social, organizational, and financial barriers to holistic care for individuals, population groups, and communities and working to eliminate these barriers while balancing justice with compassion

  - Sharing knowledge and understanding of a wide range of cultural norms and healthcare practices/beliefs/values concerning individuals, families, groups, and communities from varied racial, ethnic, spiritual, and social backgrounds

Continued ▶

- Acting as a leader, collaborator, consultant, and change agent in evaluating global health issues and environmental safety, anticipating the potential effect of environmental hazards on the health or welfare of individuals, groups, and communities, and assisting in reducing or eliminating environmental hazards

Glossary

Allopathic/conventional therapies. Medical, surgical, pharmacological, and invasive and noninvasive diagnostic procedures; those interventions most commonly used in allopathic, Western medicine.

Complementary/alternative modalities (CAM). A broad set of healthcare practices, therapies, and modalities that address the whole person—body, mind, emotion, spirit—not just signs and symptoms, that can replace or may be used as complements to conventional Western medical, surgical, and pharmacological treatments.

Critical thinking. An active, purposeful, organized cognitive process involving creativity, reflection, problem-solving, both rational and intuitive judgment, attitude of inquiry, and a philosophical orientation toward thinking about thinking.

Cultural competence. The ability to deliver health care with knowledge of and sensitivity to cultural factors that influence the health behavior, curing, healing, dying, and the grieving process of the person.

Environment. The context of habitat within which all living systems participate and interact, including the physical body and its physical habitat along with the cultural, psychological, social, and historical influences; includes both the external physical space and the person's internal physical, mental, emotional, social, and spiritual experience.

Evidence-based practice. The process by which integrative healthcare practitioners make clinical decisions using the best integrative philosophy and theories, research evidence, clinical expertise, and patient preferences within the context of available resources.

Healing. A lifelong journey into wholeness, seeking harmony and balance in one's own life and in family, community, and global relations. Healing involves those physical, mental, social, and spiritual processes of recovery, repair, renewal, and transformation that increase wholeness and often (though not invariably) order and coherence. Healing is an emergent process of the whole system bringing together aspects of one's self and the body-mind-emotion-spirit-environment at deeper levels of inner knowing, leading toward integration and balance, with each aspect having equal importance and value. Healing can lead to more complex levels of personal understanding and meaning, and may be synchronous but not synonymous with curing.

Healing process. A continual journey of changing and evolving of one's self through life that is characterized by the awareness of patterns that support or that are challenges/barriers to health and healing and that may be done alone or in a healing community.

Healing relationships. The quality and characteristics of interactions between one who facilitates healing and the person in the process of healing. Characteristics of such interactions involve empathy, caring, love, warmth, trust, confidence, credibility, competence, honesty, courtesy, respect, sharing expectations, and good communication.

Healing system. A true healthcare system in which people can receive adequate, nontoxic, and noninvasive assistance in maintaining wellness and healing for body, mind, emotion, and spirit, together with the most sophisticated, aggressive curing technologies available.

Health. An individually defined state or process in which the individual (nurse, client, family, group, or community) experiences a sense of well-being, harmony, and unity such that subjective experiences about health, health beliefs, and values are honored; a process of becoming an expanding consciousness.

Health promotion. Activities and preventive measures to promote health, increase well-being, and actualize human potential of people, families, communities, society, and ecology such as immunizations, fitness/exercise programs, breast self-exam, appropriate nutrition, relaxation, stress management, social support, prayer, meditation, healing rituals, cultural practices, and promoting environmental health and safety.

Holistic communication. A free flow of verbal and nonverbal interchange between and among people and significant beings such as pets, nature, and God/Life Force/Absolute/Transcendent that explores meaning and ideas leading to mutual understanding and growth.

Holistic ethics. The basic underlying concept of the unity and integral wholeness of all people and of all nature, identified and pursued by finding unity and wholeness within the self and within humanity. In this framework, acts are not performed for the sake of law, precedent, or social norms, but rather from a desire to do good freely in order to witness, identify, and contribute to unity.

Holistic healing. A form of healing based on attention to all aspects of an individual: physical, mental, emotional, sexual, cultural, social, and spiritual.

Holistic nurse. A nurse who recognizes and integrates body-mind-emotion-spirit-environment principles and modalities in daily life and clinical practice, creates a caring healing space within herself/himself that allows the nurse to be an instrument of healing, shares authenticity of unconditional presence that helps to remove the barriers to the healing process, facilitates another person's growth (body-mind-emotion-spirit-environment connections), and assists with recovery from illness or transition to peaceful death.

Holistic nursing practice process. An iterative and integrative process that involves six steps that may occur simultaneously: (1) assessing, (2) diagnosing or identifying patterns/challenges/needs/health issue(s), (3) identifying outcomes, (4) planning care, (5) implementing the plan of care, and (6) evaluating.

Honor. An act or intention indicating the holding of self or another in high respect, esteem, and dignity, including valuing and accepting the humanity of people, with regard for the decisions and wishes of another.

Human caring. The moral ideal of nursing in which the nurse brings one's whole self into a relationship with the whole self of the person being cared for in order to protect that person's vulnerability, preserve her or his humanity and dignity, and reinforce the meaning and experience of oneness and unity.

Human health experience. That totality of human experience including each person's subjective experience about health, health beliefs, values, sexual orientation, and personal preferences that encompasses health-wellness-disease-illness-death.

Illness. A subjective experience of symptoms and suffering to which the individual ascribes meaning and significance; not synonymous with disease; a shift in the homeodynamic balance of the person.

Intention. The conscious awareness of being in the present moment to help facilitate the healing process; a volitional act of love.

Interdisciplinary. Conversation or collaboration across disciplines where knowledge is shared that informs learning, practice, education, and research; it includes individuals, families, community members, and other disciplines.

Meaning. That which is signified, indicated, referred to, or understood. More specifically: *Philosophical meaning* – Meaning that depends on the symbolic connections that are grasped by reason. *Psychological meaning* – Meaning that depends on connections that are experienced through intuition or insight.

Person. An individual, client, patient, family member, support person, or community member who has the opportunity to engage in interaction with a holistic nurse.

Person-centered care. The human caring process in which the holistic nurse gives full attention and intention to the whole self of a person, not merely the current presenting symptoms, illness, crisis, or tasks to be accomplished, and that includes reinforcing the person's meaning and experience of oneness and unity; the condition of trust that is created in which holistic care can be given and received.

Presence. The essential state or core in healing; approaching an individual in a way that respects and honors her/his essence; relating in a way that reflects a quality of being with and in collaboration with rather than doing to; entering into a shared experience (or field of consciousness) that promotes healing potential and an experience of well-being.

Relationship-centered care. A process model of caregiving that is based in a vision of community where three types of relationships are identified: (1) patient–practitioner relationship, (2) community–practitioner relationship, and (3) practitioner–practitioner relationship. Each of these interrelated relationships is essential within a reformed integrative healthcare delivery system in a hospital, clinic, community, or in the home. Each component involves a unique set of responsibilities and tasks that addresses three areas: knowledge, values, and skills (Tresolini & Pew-Fetzer 1994).

Spirituality. The feelings, thoughts, experiences, and behaviors that arise from a search for meaning. That which is generally considered sacred or holy. Usually, though not universally, considered to involve a sense of connection with an absolute, imminent, or transcendent spiritual force, however named, as well as the conviction that meaning, value, direction, and purpose are valid aspects of the individual and universe.

The essence of being and relatedness that permeates all of life and is manifested in one's knowing, doing, and being. The interconnectedness with self, others, nature, and God/Life Force/Absolute/Transcendent. Not necessarily synonymous with religion.

Transpersonal. A personal understanding that is based on one's experiences of temporarily transcending or moving beyond one's usual identification with the limited biological, historical, cultural, and personal self at the deepest and most profound levels of experience possible. From this perspective the ordinary, biological, historical, cultural, and personal self is seen as an important but only a partial manifestation or expression of this much greater something that is one's deeper origin and destination. That which transcends the limits and boundaries of individual ego identities and possibilities to include acknowledgment and appreciation of something greater.

Wellness. Integrated, congruent functioning aimed toward reaching one's highest potential.

(Most of the definitions in this document were adapted from Dossey et al. 2005, with permission, and AHNA's *Standards of Holistic Nursing Practice*, 2005.)

REFERENCES

American Association of Colleges of Nursing. (1996). *The essentials of master's education for advanced practice nursing.* Washington, DC: AACN.

American Holistic Nurses Association. (1998). *Description of holistic nursing.* Flagstaff, AZ: AHNA.

American Holistic Nurses Association. (2005). *Standards of holistic nursing practice.* Flagstaff, AZ: AHNA.

American Holistic Nurses Association. (2005). *Standards of advanced holistic nursing practice for graduate-prepared nurses.* Flagstaff, AZ: AHNA.

American Holistic Nurses Association. (2007). *Position statement on holistic nursing ethics.* Flagstaff, AZ: AHNA.

American Nurses Association. (1996). *Scope and standards of advanced practice registered nursing practice.* Washington, DC: American Nurses Publishing.

American Nurses Association. (2001). *Code of ethics for nurses with interpretive statements.* Washington, DC: American Nurses Publishing.

American Nurses Association. (2003). *Nursing's social policy statement, 2nd ed.* Silver Spring, MD: Nursesbooks.org.

American Nurses Association. (2004). *Nursing: Scope and standards of practice.* Silver Spring, MD: Nursesbooks.org.

Barnes, P.M., E. Powell-Griner, K. McFann, & R.L. Nahin. (2004). Complementary and alternative medicine use among adults: United States, 2002. *Advance data from vital and health statistics*, No. 243, May 27, 2004. Hyattsville, MD: U.S. Department of Health and Human Services, Center for Disease Control and Prevention, and National Center for

Alternative and Complementary Medicine. (Available online: http://www.mbcrc.med.ucla.edu/PDFs/camsurvey2.pdf)

Dossey, B., L. Keagan, & C. Guzzetta. (2005). *Holistic nursing: A handbook for practice, 4th ed.* Sudbury, MA: Jones and Bartlett.

Eisenberg, D.M., R. C. Kessler, C. Foster, F. E. Norlock, D.R. Calkins, & T. L. Delbanco. (1993). Unconventional medicine in the United States: Prevalence, costs, and patterns of use. *New England Journal of Medicine* 328(4): 246–252. (Abstract and citations available online: http://content.nejm.org/cgi/content/short/328/4/246)

Eisenberg, D., R. B. Davis, S. L. Ettner, S. Appel, S. Wiilke, M. Van Rompay, & R. C. Kessler. (1998). Trends in alternative medicine use in the United States, 1990–1997. *Journal of the American Medical Association* 280: 1569–75.

Eliopoulos, C. (2005). *Nurse competency in aging: Safe integration of complementary and alternative therapies in geriatric care.* Flagstaff, AZ: American Holistic Nurses Association.

Fenton, M. and D. Morris. (2003). The integration of holistic nursing practices and complementary and alternative modalities into curricula of schools of nursing. *Alternative Therapies in Health and Nursing* 9 (4): 62–67.

Frisch, N., B. Dossey, C. Guzzetta, and J. Quinn. (2000). *Standards of holistic nursing practice with guidelines for caring and healing.* Gaithersburg, MD: Aspen.

Guzzetta, C., ed. (1998). *Essential readings in holistic nursing.* Gaithersburg, MD: Aspen.

Health Forum. (2006). *Report of hospitals using complementary and alternative medicine.* Chicago: American Hospital Association.

Institute of Medicine. (2005). *Complementary and alternative medicine in the United States.* Washington, DC: The National Academies Press.

Mariano, C. (2003). Advanced practice in holistic nursing, in *Nurse practitioners: Evolution of advanced practice, 4th ed.*, ed. M. Mezey, D. McGivern, & E. Sullivan-Marx, pp. 233–253. NY: Springer Publishing Company.

National Center for Complementary and Alternative Medicine. (2005). *Expanding horizons of health care: Strategic plan 2005–2009.* Washington, DC: National Institutes of Health.

National Institute of Health. (2000). *Expanding horizons of health care (2001–2005): National Center for Complementary & Alternative Medicine's Five-Year Strategic Plan.* Bethesda, MD: NIH.

Shelky, M. (2005). *Nurse competency in aging. Aging with chronicity: Overview and resources.* Flagstaff, AZ: American Holistic Nurses Association.

Sparber, A. (2001). State boards of nursing and scope of practice of registered nurses performing complementary therapies. *Online Journal of Issues in Nursing,* 6(3), Manuscript 10. Retrieved from http://www.nursingworld.org/ojin/topic15/tpc15_6.htm

Tresolini, C.P., & Pew-Fetzer Task Force. (1994). *Health professions education and relationship-centered care: Report of the Pew-Fetzer Task Force on advancing psychosocial health education.* San Francisco, CA: Pew Health Professions Commission. (Available online at http://www.futurehealth.ucsf.edu/pdf_files/RelationshipCentered.pdf)

U.S. Department of Health and Human Services. (1999a). *The patients' bill of rights in Medicare and Medicaid.* Accessed on January 1, 2007, at http://www.hhs.gov/news/press/1999pres/990412.html

U.S. Department of Health and Human Services. (1999b). *National health interview survey 1999.* Center for Disease Control and Prevention. National Center for Health Statistics. Division of Health Interview Statistics. Hyattsville. MD: U.S. DHHS.

U.S. Department of Health and Human Services. (2005). *Healthy People 2010 Midcourse review.* U.S. DHHS 2005. Available online at http://www.healthypeople.gov/data/midcourse/default.htm

Watson, J. (2005). *Caring science as sacred science*. Philadelphia: F.A. Davis.

Weeks, J. (2001). Foreword, in *Mosby's complementary and alternative medicine: A research-based approach,* eds. L. W. Freeman & G. F. Lawlis. St. Louis: Mosby.

White House Commission on Complementary and Alternative Medicine Policy (WHCCAMP). (2001). Interim progress report. *Alternative Therapies in Health and Medicine* 7(6): 32–40.

White House Commission on Complementary and Alternative Medicine Policy (WHCCAMP). (2002). *Final report*. Washington, DC: U.S. Government Printing Office.

BIBLIOGRAPHY

American Holistic Nurses Association. (2005). *Standards of holistic nursing practice*. Flagstaff, AZ: AHNA. (Included as Appendix B in this book starting, on page 81)

American Holistic Nurses Association. (2005). *Standards of advanced holistic nursing practice for graduate prepared nurses*. Flagstaff, AZ: AHNA. (Included as Appendix C in this book, starting on page 93)

American Holistic Nurses Association (2007). *Position on nursing research and scholarship*. Flagstaff, AZ: AHNA.

American Holistic Nurses Association. (2007). *Position on the role of nurses in the practice of complementary and alternative therapies*. Flagstaff, AZ: AHNA.

Dossey, B., ed. (1997). *Core curriculum for holistic nursing*. Gaithersburg, MD: Aspen.

Dossey, B., L. Keagan, and C. Guzzetta. (2005). *Holistic nursing: A handbook for practice, 4th ed*. Gaithersburg, MD: Aspen.

Frisch, N., B. Dossey, C. Guzzetta, and J. Quinn. (2000). AHNA *standards of holistic nursing practice: Guidelines for caring and healing*. Gaithersburg, MD: Aspen.

Guzzetta, C., ed. (1998). *Essential readings in holistic nursing*. Gaithersburg, MD: Aspen.

Mariano, C. (2003). Advanced practice in holistic nursing, in *Nurse practitioners: Evolution of advanced practice, 4th ed*., eds. M. Mezey, D. McGivern, & E. Sullivan-Marx. NY: Springer Publishing Company.

Mariano, C. (2005). An overview of holistic nursing. *Imprint* 52 (2): 1148–52.

Watson, J. (2004). *Caring science as sacred science*. Philadelphia: F.A. Davis.

Appendix A
Categories of Complementary/Alternative Modalities (CAM) Therapies

In the context of this book, these descriptive categories encompass generally but not exhaustively those therapies described as alternative or complementary. (See also the CAM Glossary entry on page 67.)

Biologically based therapies. Biologically based therapies in CAM use substances found in nature, such as herbs, food, vitamins, minerals, and botanicals. Some examples include herbal products, dietary supplements, whole diet therapies, and Aromatherapy.

Energy therapies. Energy therapies involve the use of the energy fields. They are two types:

Bioelectromagnetic-based therapies. Involve the unconventional use of electromagnetic fields, such as pulse fields, magnetic fields, or alternating-current or direct-current fields.

Biofield therapies. Intended to affect energy fields that purportedly surround and penetrate the human body. Includes acupuncture. Some forms of energy therapy manipulate biofields by applying pressure, e.g., acupressure and/or manipulating the body by placing the hands in or through these fields. Examples include Qi Gong, Reiki, Therapeutic Touch, and Healing Touch.

Manipulative and body-based methods. Manipulative and body-based methods in CAM are based on manipulation and/or movement of one or more parts of the body. Some examples include Chiropractic or Osteopathic manipulation, massage, Trager Body Work, Reflexology, Crainal-Sacral, Rolfing, Alexander Technique, Feldenkrais Technique, Polarity, and Pilates.

Mind–body interventions. Mind–body medicine uses a variety of techniques designed to enhance the mind's capacity to affect bodily function and symptoms. Some techniques that were considered CAM in the past have become mainstream (for example, patient support groups, psychotherapy, cognitive-behavioral therapy). Other mind–body techniques are meditation, relaxation, imagery, hypnosis, yoga, biofeedback, Tai Chi, autogenic training, spirituality, prayer, mental healing, and therapies that use creative outlets such as art, music, dance, or journaling.

Whole medical systems. Alternative medical systems are built upon complete systems of theory and practice. Often, these systems have evolved apart from and earlier than the conventional medical approach used in the United States. Examples of Whole medical systems that have developed in Western cultures include Homeopathic medicine and Naturopathic medicine. Examples of systems that have developed in non-Western cultures include Traditional Chinese medicine and Ayurvedic medicine (India). Some Traditional Indigenous healing systems include Native American, African, Middle Eastern, Tibetan, Central and South American, and Curanderismo.

Source: National Center for Complementary and Alternative Medicine, National Institutes of Health and Human Services, 2007. http:// nccam.nih.gov

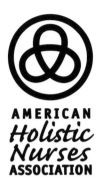

APPENDIX B

American Holistic Nurses Association

Standards of Holistic Nursing Practice

Revised 2005

AMERICAN
Holistic
Nurses
ASSOCIATION

Contents

Acknowledgements

AHNA Task Force Co-Chairpersons

Barbara Montgomery Dossey, MS, RN, HNC, FAAN; Noreen Cavan Frisch, PhD, RN, HNC, FAAN

AHNA Task Force Committee Members

Cathie E. Guzzetta, PhD, RN, HNC, FAAN; Lynn Keegan, PhD, RN, HNC, FAAN; Susan Luck, MA, RN, HNC; Johanne A. Quinn, PhD, RN, HNC; Lynn Rew, EdD, RN, HNC, FAAN; Louise C. Selanders, EdD, RN

Advisory Committee Members

Mary E. Brekke, PhD, RN, HNC, CHTP; Joanne Evans, MEd, RN, CS, HNC; Kathleen Fasnacht, MA, MSN, ARNPC, HNC; Cheryl Hann, RN, HNC; Sharron Harcarik, MS, RN, HNC; Rhonda Kantor, BSN, BS, RN, HNC; Judy M. Kaplan, BS, RN, CCRC, HNC; Kathryn Keegan, RNC, HNC, CHTP; JoAnn Glittenberg Kropp, PhD, RN, HNC, FAAN; Bonnie Mackey, MSN, ARNP, CMT, HNC; Peggy Moses, MS, RN, MSN; Sharon Murnane, BA(c), RN, HNC, CHTP; Joyce O. Murphy, BS, RN, HNC; Laurie Murphy, BSN, RN, HNC; Bobbie Nisbet, RN, HNC, CHTP; Nancy Oliver, PhD, RN, HNC; Clark S. Roberts, RN, HNC, CMT, CHTP; Sonja Simpson, MSN, RN; Patricia R. Skidmore, MSN, RN, HNC; Susanna Smart, BSN, RN, CRT, CMT, CCHT, CRBP, HNC; Pina Sperber, BSN, RN; Diane J. Urban, MS, RNC, NP, HNC; Christine B. Ussard, BSN, RN, HNC; Gretchen Wiederrecht, MS, RN, HNC

Review Committee

Jeanne Anselmo, BSN, RN, HNC; Elizabeth Ann Manhart Barrett, PhD, RN, FAAN; Genevieve M. Bartol, EdD, RN, HNC; Margaret A. Burkhardt, PhD, RN, CS, HNC; Nancy Fleming Courts, PhD, RN, NCC; Joan Engebretson, DrPH, RN, HNC; Kimetha S. Falkenburg, BSN, RN; Lea Barbato Gaydos, PhD, MSN, RN, CS, HNC; Dorothea Hover-Kramer, EdD, RN; Pamela J. Potter Hughes, MSN, RNCS, CHTP/I; Mary Gail Nagai Jacobson, MSN, RN; Karen Kauffeld, RN; Cheryl Demerath Learn, PhD, RN; Maggie McKivergin, MS, RN, CNS, HNC; Melodie Olson, PhD, RN; B.H. Rose, MEd, MSN, RN; Bonney Gulino Schaub, MS, CS; Eleanor A. Schuster, DNSc, RN, HNC; Eileen M. Stuart, RN, MS; Leona Weiner, EdD, RN, HNC; Carol L. Wells-Federman, MS, MEd, RN, CS; Wendy Wetzel, MSN, RN, FNP, HNC; Patty Wooten, BSN, RN; Christine A. Wynd, PhD, RN

Guidelines

The AHNA Standards of Holistic Nursing Practice:
- are used in conjunction with the American Nurses Association Standards of Practice and the specific specialty standards where holistic nurses practice.
- contain five core values that are followed by a description and standards of practice action statements. Depending on the setting or area of practice, holistic nurses may or may not use all of these actions statements.
- draw on modalities derived from a number of explanatory models, of which biomedicine is only one model.
- reflect the diverse nursing activities in which holistic nurses are engaged.
- serve holistic nurses in personal life, clinical and private practice, education, research, and community service.

AHNA Holistic Nursing Practice Definitions

Allopathic/Traditional Therapies: medical, surgery, invasive and noninvasive diagnostic treatment procedures, including medications.

Caring-Healing Interventions: nontraditional therapies that can interface with traditional medical and surgical therapies; may be used as complements to conventional medical and surgical treatments; also called alternative/complementary/integrative therapies or interventions. See list of interventions most frequently used in holistic nursing practice.

Client of Holistic Nursing: an individual, family, group, or community of persons who is engaged in interactions with a holistic nurse in a manner respectful of each client's subjective experience about health, health beliefs, values, sexual orientation, and personal preferences.

Cultural Competence: the ability to deliver health care with knowledge of and sensitivity to cultural factors that influence the health behavior of the person.

Environment: everything that surrounds the person, both the external and the internal (physical, mental, emotional, and spiritual) environment as well as patterns not yet understood.

Healing: the process of bringing together aspects of one's self, body-mind-spirit, at deeper levels of inner knowing leading toward integration and balance with each aspect having equal importance and value; can lead to more complex levels of personal understanding and meaning; may be synchronous but not synonymous with curing.

Healing Process: a continual journey of changing and evolving of one's self through life; the awareness of patterns that support or are challenges/barriers to health and healing; may be done alone or in a healing community.

Health: the state or process in which the individual (nurse, client, family, group, or community) experiences a sense of well-being, harmony, and unity where subjective experiences about health, health beliefs, and values are honored.

Health Promotion: activities and preventive measures such as immunizations, fitness/exercise programs, breast self exam, appropriate nutrition, relaxation, stress management, social support, prayer, meditation, healing rituals, cultural practices, and promoting environmental health and safety.

Holistic Caring Process: a circular process that involves six steps which may occur simultaneously. These parts are assessment, patterns/challenges/needs, outcomes, therapeutic care plan, implementation, and evaluation.

Holistic Communication: a free flow of verbal and nonverbal interchange between and among people and significant beings such as pets, nature, and God/Life Force/Absolute/Transcendent that explores meaning and ideas leading to mutual understanding and growth.

Holistic Nurse: a nurse who recognizes and integrates body-mind-spirit principles and modalities in daily life and clinical practice; one who creates a healing space within herself/himself that allows the nurse to be an instrument of healing for the purpose of helping another feel safe and more in harmony; one who shares authenticity of unconditional presence that help to remove the barriers to the healing process.

Human Caring Process: the moral state in which the holistic nurse brings her or his whole self into relationship to the whole self of significant beings which reinforces the meaning and experience of oneness and unity.

Intention: the conscious awareness of being in the present moment to help facilitate the healing process; a volitional act of love.

Intuition: perceived knowing of things and events without the conscious use of rational processes; using all the senses to receive information.

Patterns/Challenges/Needs: a person's actual and potential life processes related to health, wellness, disease, or illness which may or may not facilitate well-being.

Person: an individual, client, patient, family member, support person, or community member who has the opportunity to engage in interaction with a holistic nurse.

Person-Centered Care: the condition of trust that is created where holistic care can be given and received; the human caring process in which the holistic nurse gives full attention and intention to the whole self of a person, not merely the current presenting symptoms, illness, crisis, or tasks to be accomplished; reinforcing the person's meaning and experience of oneness and unity.

Presence: the essential state or core in healing; approaching an individual in a way that respects and honors her/his essence; relating in a way that reflects a quality of *being with* and *in collaboration with* rather than *doing to*; entering into a shared experience (or field of consciousness) that promotes healing potentials and an experience of well-being.

Spirituality: a unifying force of a person; the essence of being that permeates all of life and is manifested in one's being, knowing, and doing; the interconnectedness with self, others, nature, and God/Life Force/ Absolute/ Transcendent.

Standards of Practice: a group of statements describing the expected level of care by a holistic nurse.

AHNA Holistic Nursing Description

Holistic nursing embraces all nursing which has enhancement of healing the whole person from birth to death as its goal. Holistic nursing recognizes that there are two views regarding holism: that holism involves identifying the interrelationships of the bio-psycho-social-spiritual dimensions of the person, recognizing that the whole is greater than the sum of its parts; and that holism involves understanding the individual as a unitary whole in mutual process with the environment. Holistic nursing responds to both views, believing that the goals of nursing can be achieved within either framework.

The holistic nurse is an instrument of healing and a facilitator in the healing process. Holistic nurses honor the individual's subjective experience about health, health beliefs, and values. To become therapeutic partners with individuals, families, and communities, holistic nursing practice draws on nursing knowledge, theories, research, expertise, intuition, and creativity. Holistic nursing practice encourages peer review of professional practice in various clinical settings and integrates knowledge of current professional standards, laws, and regulations governing nursing practice.

Practicing holistic nursing requires nurses to integrate self-care, self-responsibility, spirituality, and reflection in their lives. This may lead the nurse to greater awareness of the interconnectedness with self, others, nature, and God/LifeForce/Absolute/ Transcendent. This awareness may further enhance the nurses' understanding of all individuals and their relationships to the human and global community, and permits nurses to use this awareness to facilitate the healing process.

Interventions Most Frequently Used In Holistic Nursing Practice[1]

Acupressure	Healing Presence	Play Therapy
Aromatherapy	Healing Touch Modalities	Prayer
Art Therapy	Holistic Self-Assessments	Reflexology
Biofeedback	Humor and Laughter	Relaxation Modalities
Cognitive Therapy	Journaling	Self-Care Interventions
Counseling[2]	Massage	Self-Reflection
Exercise and Movement	Meditation	Smoking Cessation
Goal-Setting and Contracts	Music and Sound Therapy	Therapeutic Touch
Guided Imagery	Nutrition Counseling	Weight Management

1   See Dossey, B., Frisch, N., Forker, J., and Lavin, J. Evolving a Blueprint for Certification: Inventory of Professional Activities and Knowledge of a Holistic Nurse, *Journal of Holistic Nursing*, 1998, Vol. 16, No. 1, p 33—56.
2   Used in situations such as addictions, death and grief; unhealthy environments, relationship issues, sexual abuse, spiritual needs, violence, support groups, wellness promotion, and life-style issues.

Summary of AHNA Core Values

CORE VALUE 1: Holistic Philosophy, Theories, and Ethics
Holistic nursing practice is based on the philosophy and theory of holism and the foundation of ethical practice.

   1.1   **Holistic Philosophy.** Holistic nurses develop and expand their conceptual framework and overall philosophy in the art and science of holistic nursing to effectively model, practice, teach, and conduct research.

   1.2   **Holistic Theories.** Nursing theories that are holistic, and other relevant theories, provide the framework for all aspects of holistic nursing practice and leadership.

   1.3   **Holistic Ethics.** Holistic nurses hold to a professional ethic of caring and healing that seeks to preserve wholeness and dignity of themselves and all persons/families/communities in all practice settings.

CORE VALUE 2: Holistic Education and Research
Holistic nursing practice is guided by, and developed through, holistic education and research.

   2.1   **Holistic Education.** Holistic nurses acquire and maintain current knowledge and competency in holistic nursing practice.

   2.2   **Holistic Research.** Holistic nurses provide care and guidance to persons through nursing interventions and holistic therapies consistent with research findings and other sound evidence.

CORE VALUE 3: Holistic Nurse Self-Care
Holistic nursing practice requires the integration of self-care and personal development activities into one's life.

   3.1   **Holistic Nurse Self-Care.** Holistic nurses engage in holistic self-assessment, self-care, and personal development, aware of being instruments of healing to better serve self and others.

CORE VALUE 4: Holistic Communication, Therapeutic Environment, and Cultural Diversity
Holistic nursing practice honors and includes holistic communication, therapeutic environment, and cultural diversity as foundational concepts.

   4.1   **Holistic Communication.** Holistic nurses engage in holistic communication to ensure that each person experiences the presence of the nurse as authentic and sincere; there is an atmosphere of shared humanness that includes a sense of connectedness and attention reflecting the individual's uniqueness.

   4.2   **Therapeutic Environment.** Holistic nurses recognize that each person's environment includes everything within and surrounding the individual, as well as patterns not yet understood.

   4.3   **Cultural Diversity.** Holistic nurses recognize each person as a whole body-mind-emotion-spirit being and mutually create a plan of care consistent with cultural background, health beliefs and practices, sexual orientation, values, and preferences.

CORE VALUE 5: Holistic Caring Process
Holistic nursing practice is guided by the holistic caring process, whether used with individuals, families, population groups, or communities. This circular process involves the following six steps, which may occur simultaneously.

   5.1   **Assessment.** Holistic nurses assess each person holistically using appropriate conventional and holistic methods while the uniqueness of the person is honored.

   5.2   **Patterns/Challenges/Needs.** Holistic nurses identify and prioritize each person's actual and potential patterns/ challenges/ needs and life processes related to health, wellness, disease, or illness, which may or may not facilitate well-being.

   5.3   **Outcomes.** Holistic nurses specify appropriate outcomes for each person's actual or potential patterns/challenges/ needs.

   5.4   **Therapeutic Care Plans.** Holistic nurses engage each person to mutually create an appropriate plan of care that focuses on health promotion, recovery, restoration, or peaceful dying so that the person is as independent as possible.

   5.5   **Implementation.** Holistic nurses prioritize each person's plan of holistic care, and holistic nursing interventions are implemented accordingly.

   5.6   **Evaluation.** Holistic nurses evaluate each person's response to holistic care regularly and systematically and the continuing holistic nature of the healing process is recognized and honored.

CORE VALUE 1: Holistic Philosophy, Theories, and Ethics

Holistic nursing practice is based on the philosophy and theory of holism and the foundation of ethical practice.

1.1 Holistic Philosophy
Holistic nurses develop and expand their conceptual framework and overall philosophy in the art and science of holistic nursing to model, practice, teach, and conduct research in the most effective manner possible.

Standards of Practice
Holistic nurses:

1.1.1   recognize the person's capacity for self-healing and the importance of supporting the natural development and unfolding of that capacity.

1.1.2   support, share, and recognize expertise and competency in holistic nursing practice that is used in many diverse clinical and community settings.

1.1.3   participate in person-centered care by being a partner, coach, and mentor who actively listens and supports others in reaching personal goals.

1.1.4   focus on strategies to bring harmony, unity, and healing to the nursing profession.

1.1.5   communicate with traditional health care practitioners about appropriate referrals to other holistic practitioners when needed.

1.1.6   interact with professional organizations in a leadership or membership capacity at local, state, national, and international levels to further expand the knowledge and practice of holistic nursing and awareness of holistic health issues.

1.2 Holistic Theories.
Nursing theories that are holistic, and other relevant theories, provide the framework for all aspects of holistic nursing practice and leadership.

Standards of Practice
Holistic nurses:

1.2.1   strive to use nursing theories to develop holistic nursing practice and transformational leadership.

1.2.2   interpret, use, and document information relevant to a person's care according to a theoretical framework.

1.3 Holistic Ethics
Holistic nurses hold to a professional ethic of caring and healing that seeks to preserve wholeness an dignity of themselves and all persons/families/communities in all practice settings.

Standards of Practice
Holistic nurses:

1.3.1   identify the ethics of caring and its contribution to unity of self, others, nature, and God/Life Force/Absolute/Transcendent as central to holistic nursing practice.

1.3.2   integrate the standards of holistic nursing practice with applicable state laws and regulations governing nursing practice.

1.3.3   engage in activities that respect, nurture, and enhance the integral relationship with the earth, and advocate for the well-being of the global community's economy, education, and social justice.

1.3.4   advocate for the rights of patients to have educated choices into their plan of care.

1.3.5   participate in peer evaluation to ensure knowledge and competency in holistic nursing practice.

1.3.6   protect the personal privacy and confidentiality of individuals, especially with health care agencies and managed care organizations.

CORE VALUE 2: Holistic Education and Research

Holistic nursing practice is guided by, and developed through, holistic education and research.

2.1 Holistic Education
Holistic nurses acquire and maintain current knowledge and competency in holistic nursing practice.

Standards of Practice
Holistic nurses:
- 2.1.1   participate in activities of continuing education and related fields that have relevance to holistic nursing practice.
- 2.1.2   identify areas of knowledge from nursing and various fields such as biomedical, epidemiology, behavioral medicine, cultural and social theories.
- 2.1.3   continually develop and standardize holistic nursing guidelines, protocols and practice to promote competency in holistic nursing practice and assure quality of care to individuals.
- 2.1.4   use the results of quality care activities to initiate change in holistic nursing practice.
- 2.1.5   may seek certification in holistic nursing as one means of advancing the philosophy and practice of holistic nursing.

2.2 Holistic Nursing and Related Research
Holistic nurses provide care and guidance to persons through nursing interventions and holistic therapies consistent with research findings and other sound evidence.

Standards of Practice
Holistic nurses:
- 2.2.1   use available research and evidence from different explanatory models to mutually create a plan of care with a person.
- 2.2.2   use expert clinical judgment to select appropriate interventions.
- 2.2.3   discuss holistic application to clinical situations where rigorous research has not been done.
- 2.2.4   create an environment conducive to systematic inquiry into healing and health issues by engaging in research or supporting and utilizing the research of others.
- 2.2.5   disseminate research findings at meetings and through publications to further develop the foundation and practice of holistic nursing.
- 2.2.6   provide consultation services on holistic nursing interventions to persons and communities based on research.

CORE VALUE 3: Holistic Nurse Self-Care

Holistic nursing practice requires the integration of self-care and personal development activities into one's life.

3.1 Holistic Nurse Self-Care
Holistic nurses engage in holistic self-assessment, self-care, and personal development, aware of being instruments of healing to better serve self and others.

Standards of Practice
Holistic nurses:

3.1.1 recognize that a person's body-mind-spirit has healing capacities that can be enhanced and supported through self-care practices.

3.1.2 identify and integrate self-care strategies to enhance their physical, psychological, sociological, and spiritual well-being.

3.1.3 recognize and address at-risk health patterns and begin the process of change.

3.1.4 consciously cultivate awareness and understanding about the deeper meaning, purpose, inner strengths, and connection with self, others, nature, and God/Life Force/Absolute/Transcendent.

3.1.5 use clear intention to care for self and to seek a sense of balance, harmony, and joy in daily life.

3.1.6 participate in the evolutionary holistic process with the understanding that crisis creates opportunity in any setting.

CORE VALUE 4: Holistic Communication, Therapeutic Environment, and Cultural Diversity

Holistic nursing practice honors and includes holistic communication, therapeutic environment, and cultural diversity as foundational concepts.

4.1 Holistic Communication
Holistic nurses engage in holistic communication to ensure that each person experiences the presence of the nurse as authentic and sincere; there is an atmosphere of shared humanness that includes a sense of connectedness and attention reflecting the individual's uniqueness.

Standards of Practice
Holistic nurses:

4.1.1　develop an awareness of the most frequently encountered challenges to holistic communication.

4.1.2　increase therapeutic and cultural competence skills to enhance their effectiveness through listening to themselves and others.

4.1.3　explore with each person those strategies that can assist her/him, as desired, to understand the deeper meaning, purpose, inner strengths, and connections with self, others, nature, and God/Life Force/Absolute/Transcendent.

4.1.4　recognize that holistic communication and awareness of individuals is a continuously evolving multi-level exchange that offers itself through dreams, images, symbols, sensations, meditations, and prayers.

4.1.5　respect the person's health trajectory which may be incongruent with conventional wisdom.

4.2 Therapeutic Environment
Holistic nurses recognize that each person's environment includes everything that surrounds the individual, both the external and the internal (physical, mental, emotional, and spiritual) as well as patterns not yet understood.

Standards of Practice
Holistic nurses:

4.2.1　promote environments conducive to experiencing healing, wholeness and harmony, and care for the person in as healthy an environment as possible.

4.2.2　work toward creating organizations that value sacred space and environments that enhance healing.

4.2.3　integrate holistic principles, standards, policies and procedures in relation to environmental safety and emergency preparedness.

4.2.4　recognize that the well-being of the ecosystem of the planet is a prior determining condition for the well-being of the human.

4.2.5　promote social networks and social environments where healing can take place.

4.3 Cultural Diversity
Holistic nurses recognize each person as a whole body-mind-emotion-spirit being and mutually create a plan of care consistent with cultural background, health beliefs and practices, sexual orientation, values, and preferences.

Standards of Practice
Holistic nurses:

4.3.1　assess and incorporate the person's cultural practices, values, beliefs, meanings of health, illness, and risk behaviors in care and health education.

4.3.2　use appropriate community resources and experts to extend their understanding of different cultures.

4.3.3　assess for discriminatory practices and change as necessary.

4.3.4　identify discriminatory health care practices as they impact the person and engage in effective nondiscriminatory practices.

CORE VALUE 5: Holistic Caring Process

Holistic nursing practice is guided by the holistic caring process, whether used with individuals, families, population groups, or communities. This circular process involves the following six steps, which may occur simultaneously.

5.1 Assessment
Holistic nurses assess each person holistically using appropriate conventional and holistic methods while the uniqueness of the person is honored.

Standards of Practice
Holistic nurses:

5.1.1 use an assessment process including appropriate traditional and holistic methods to systematically gather information.

5.1.2 value all types of knowing including intuition when gathering data from a person and validate this intuitive knowledge with the person when appropriate.

5.2 Patterns/Challenges/Needs
Holistic nurses identify and prioritize each person's actual and potential patterns/challenges/needs and life processes related to health, wellness, disease, or illness, which may or may not facilitate well being.

Standards of Practice
Holistic nurses:

5.2.1 assist the person to access inner wisdom that can provide opportunities to enhance and support growth, development and movement towards health and well-being.

5.2.2 collect data and collaborate with the person and health care team members as appropriate to identify and record a list of actual and potential patterns/challenges/needs.

5.2.3 use collected data to formulate an etiology of the person's identified actual or potential patterns/challenges/needs.

5.2.4 make referrals to other holistic practitioners or traditional therapist when appropriate.

5.3 Outcomes
Holistic nurses specify appropriate outcomes for each person's actual or potential patterns/challenges/needs.

Standards of Practice
Holistic nurses:

5.3.1 honor the person in all phases of her/his healing process regardless of expectations or outcomes.

5.3.2 identify and partner with the person to specify measurable outcomes and realistic goals.

5.4 Therapeutic Care Plan
Holistic nurses engage each person to mutually create an appropriate plan of care that focuses on health promotion, recovery, restoration, or peaceful dying so that the person is as independent as possible.

Standards of Practice
Holistic nurses:

5.4.1 partner with the person in a mutual decision process to create a health care plan for each pattern/challenge/need or opportunity to enhance health and well-being.

5.4.2 help a person identify areas for education to make decisions about life choices in a conscious, informed manner that empowers the person to maintain her/his uniqueness and independence.

5.4.3 offer self-assessment tools, word associations, storytelling, dreams, journals as appropriate.

5.4.4 use skills of cultural competence and communicate acceptance of the person's values, belief, culture, religion, and socioeconomic background.

5.4.5 assist the person in recognizing at-risk patterns/challenges/needs for potential or existing health situations (e.g., personal habits, personal and family health history, age-related risk factors), and also assist in recognizing opportunities to enhance well-being.

5.4.6 engage the person in problem-solving dialogue in relation to living with changes secondary to illness and treatment.

5.5 Implementation
Holistic nurses prioritize each person's plan of holistic care, and holistic nursing interventions are implemented accordingly.

Standards of Practice
Holistic nurses:

5.5.1 implement the mutually created plan of care within the context of assisting the person towards the higher potential of health and well-being.

5.5.2 support and promote the person's capacity for the highest level of participation and problem-solving in the plan of care and collaborate with other health team members when appropriate.

5.5.3 use holistic nursing skills in implementing care including cultural competency and all ways of knowing.

5.5.4 advocate that the person's plan, choices, and unique healing journey be honored.

5.5.5 provide care that is clear about and respectful of the economic parameters of practice, balancing justice with compassion.

5.6 Evaluation
Holistic nurses evaluate each person's response to holistic care regularly and systematically and the continuing holistic nature of the healing process is recognized and honored.

Standards of Practice
Holistic nurses:

5.6.1 collaborate with the person and with other health care team members when appropriate in evaluating holistic outcomes.

5.6.2 explore with the person her/his understanding of the cause of any significant deviation between the responses and the expected outcomes.

5.6.3 mutually create with the person and other team members a revised plan if needed.

APPENDIX C

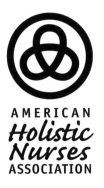

American Holistic Nurses Association

Standards of Advanced Holistic Nursing Practice for Graduate-Prepared Nurses

Revised 2005

Contents

Acknowledgements

Task Force members: Lea Barbato Gaydos, Ph.D., RN, CS, Jamie Damico, BSN, RN, LMT, Barbara Montgomery Dossey, Ph.D., R.N., HNC, FAAN, Noreen Cavan Frisch, Ph.D., RN, FAAN, HNC, Lynn Keegan, Ph.D., RN, HNC, FAAN, Cathie E. Guzzetta, Ph.D., RN, HNC, FAAN, Carla Mariano, Ed.D., RN, Johanne Quinn, Ph.D, RN, HNC, and Diane Pisanos, MS, RNC, NNP, HNC acknowledge and thank the following people involved in the review and comment on draft standards.

Responding Committee members: Anna M. Acee, Ed.D., RN, Helen Erickson, Ph.D., RN, HNC, FAAN, Joan Engebretson, Dr.Ph., RN, HNC, Lynn Rew, Ed. D., RNC, HNC, Eloise Monzillo, Ph.D., RNCS, CPHQ, Carole Schoffstall, Ph.D., RN, and Jean Watson, Ph.D., RN, FAAN, HNC.

Corresponding Committee members: Patty Aamodt, MSN, RN, CHN, Yvette Dwonch-Pena, BS, BSN, RN, Toni Gilbert, MA, RN, HNC, Donna Guyot, MS, MA, RN-CS, ANP, Linda Hein, MSN, RN, HNC, CHTP, Lucy Johnson, RN, CS, Mary Periard, Ph.D., RN, Emily Schlenker, PsyD, RN, Kim Stiles, MS, RN, HNC, Marilyn Terrado, Ph.D., RN, CS, and Arlene Wandel Zawadzki, MS, RN, CS, HNC.

Special thanks to the graduate students of Beth-El College of Nursing and Health Sciences, Colorado University, Colorado Springs, Colo., who assisted in the collation of comments on Draft 4 from all Committee and Task Force members, and Jude Fleming, BSN, RN, Lisa Wayman, BSN, RN, and Terri Woodard BSN, RN.

History of Development

In response to the growing number of graduate programs with a holistic nursing focus, the AHNA Leadership Council appointed a seven-member task force in January 2000 to develop standards for advanced practice. Two additional members joined the Task Force later that year. From that time until October 2001, the Task Force worked to develop standards for advanced holistic nursing practice. The final draft was completed and accepted for submission to the Council by the Task Force Members in September, 2001.

Meeting electronically and by telephone, the Task Force's first decision was to use the same Core Values that had been used to create the current practice standards as the foundation for developing the advanced practice standards. It was felt that regardless of the type of practice that a holistic nurse has, these values should serve as the philosophical underpinning for practice. The second decision was to use *The Essentials of Master's Education* published by the American Association of Colleges of Nursing and the *American Nurses' Association Advanced Practice Standards* as guides for the scope of practice that should be addressed by the standards since these documents are employed in the development of graduate nursing curricula. The third decision was to use essentially the same model for review of the advanced practice standards as was used to create the basic practice standards. That is, in addition to the Task Force, leaders in the field of holistic nursing and nursing education would be asked to review the draft standards to establish content validity. These leaders would form the Responding Committee and their purpose would be to make sure the standards would be congruent with national developments in graduate nursing education and holistic theory development. Over the spring, seven national holistic nursing leaders were identified and agreed to serve in this way. It was also agreed that a call should go out to the general membership asking for graduate-prepared holistic nurses with advanced practices to become members of a Corresponding Committee. The purpose of this committee would be to review the 2000 standards and provide valuable input regarding actual practice. In the July/August 2000 *Beginnings*, a call went out to the general membership asking for nurses with an advanced practice to participate. Eleven people completed the Corresponding Committee process.

A very rough Draft 1 was completed and circulated to Task Force members for review and comment in spring 2000. The comments were then used to prepare a Draft 2 for the Task Force to review at the 2000 conference in Albuquerque. At this meeting on June 9, 2000, which included the Task Force and several members of the Responding Committee, a very important decision was made. This decision was that the standards for advanced practice would apply to those nurses with a graduate degree even though there are nurses in practice with an expanded scope created not by graduate education but by certifications in particular specialties. These certifications were created before graduate education became the entry level for advanced practice. However, it was felt that the basic standards more than adequately address the scope of practice for all except graduate practice, and the need was to have standards to address holistic nursing practice by graduate-prepared nurses that would guide in the development of curricula for graduate education in holistic nursing. Several other decisions were made regarding format, organization, and content. For example, the grouping of the Core Values was slightly changed to better reflect the organization of graduate education.

During the summer of 2000, a Draft 3 was completed and circulated in the fall to Task Force members. This draft was still very rough and needed major revisions, additions, and clarifications. A Draft 4 was prepared from the feedback of Task Force members and circulated to the Responding and Corresponding Committee for review and comment. This draft was distributed to all Task Force and Committee Members March 12, 2001. An article detailing the progress of the Task Force was written and published in *Beginnings*, May-June 2001.

Comments on Draft 4 were received throughout the spring and summer of 2001. In September these comments were collated into a final draft. Draft 5, the final draft, was reviewed and accepted for submission to the Council and was mailed to the Leadership Council in October 2001. The *AHNA Standards of Advanced Holistic Nursing Practice for Graduate-Prepared Nurses* were approved and adopted by the AHNA Leadership Council in January, 2002. Minor revisions, 2004.

Introduction

The American Holistic Nurses Association (AHNA) recognizes and values the necessity of Standards of Practice to insure public safety and the provision of quality holistic care. Standards of Practice for the holistic nurse practicing at the undergraduate level have been developed and published (AHNA Standards of Holistic Nursing Practice, 2000). The proliferation of graduate programs in holistic nursing necessitates the development of standards to guide curriculum development, advanced practice, and certification at the advanced practice level.

Advanced practice education is at the graduate level, master's and doctoral. In this document the term "graduate-prepared holistic nurse" is used instead of "advanced practice holistic nurse" in each standard to acknowledge that although graduate nursing education is currently the requirement for advanced practice, many nurses have an advanced practice based on certifications beyond the basic educational level, but do not hold graduate degrees. For these nurses, the *AHNA Standards of Holistic Nursing Practice* serve as an appropriate guide to practice.

Requirements for advanced practice differ from basic nursing practice. Thus, nursing education at the graduate level has different curriculum and outcome requirements. The following *AHNA Standards of Advanced Holistic Nursing Practice for Graduate-Prepared Nurses* have been developed to be congruent with these requirements and outcomes as outlined in *The Essentials of Master's Education for Advanced Practice Nursing* (American Association of Colleges of Nursing, 1996). The following *AHNA Standards of Advanced Holistic Nursing Practice* are also congruent with the scope and standards of practice as delineated by the American Nurses Association in the *American Nurses Association Scope and Standards of Advanced Practice Registered Nursing* (ANA, 1996). Furthermore, they reflect the changing roles of the graduate-prepared nurse and the increasingly complex care environment.

Most importantly, the *American Holistic Nurses' Association Standards of Holistic Nursing Practice* (American Holistic Nurses Association, 2000) have served as the organizing framework for the *AHNA Standards of Advanced Holistic Practice for Graduate-Prepared Nurses*. Consequently, the advanced holistic practice standards proceed from the same Core Values. However, the Core Values in this document have been grouped somewhat differently than they are in the basic standards. For example, Core Value 1 is Holistic Philosophy, Theory and Ethics rather than Holistic Philosophy and Education. Core Value 2 is Holistic Education and Research rather than Holistic Ethics, Theories, and Research. These new groupings are more congruent with the way in which graduate education is organized.

Although the Core Values for these standards are essentially the same, these standards reflect a difference in the level of performance for basic nursing practice and advanced practice because the education and scope of practice is not the same. It is expected that nurses practicing at the basic level will be competent in their work. However, advanced practice indicates not only competency, but also proficiency and ultimately, expertness in the practice of holistic nursing.

Graduate-prepared nurses may or may not have prescriptive authority. The following standards are not intended to modify or replace the requirements for prescriptive authority in any Nurse Practice Act.

It is expected that graduate-prepared holistic nurses practicing at the advanced level will meet the following standards as well as the *AHNA Standards of Holistic Nursing Practice* for basic nursing practice, and standards of practice for other specialties that may apply to their practices. For example, a holistic pediatric nurse practitioner would use both the *AHNA Standards of Advanced Holistic Practice for Graduate-Prepared Nurses* and the standards of practice for pediatric nurse practitioners. For Clinical Nurse Specialists claiming holistic nursing only as their specialty, the *AHNA Standards of Advanced Holistic Practice for Graduate-Prepared Nurses* should guide practice. Educators and administrators with a holistic perspective may use the *AHNA Standards of Advanced Holistic Practice for Graduate-Prepared Nurses* to guide their work. An advanced practice certification in holistic nursing will be soon available to graduate-prepared holistic nurses who work in clinical settings, as well as nursing educators, and administrators.

Guidelines for Use

The *AHNA Standards of Advanced Holistic Practice for Graduate-Prepared Nurses* are:

used in conjunction with the *American Nurses Association Standards of Advanced Practice* and the advanced practice standards for specific specialties in which the graduate-prepared holistic nurse practices.

based on the 5 Core Values of the *AHNA Standards of Holistic Nursing Practice*. Depending on practice specialty, graduate-prepared holistic nurses may or may not use all of these action statements.

derived from a philosophy of holistic nursing, multiple theories of nursing and related fields, *The Essentials of Master's Education for Advanced Practice Nursing* published by the American Association of Colleges of Nursing (1996), biomedicine and various other models of medicine.

reflect the expanded scope and depth of knowledge required for advanced nursing practice.

appropriate as guides for the graduate-prepared holistic nurse (GPHN) in personal and professional life.

Definitions: AHNA Standards of Advanced Holistic Nursing Practice for Graduate-Prepared Nurses*

Advanced Nursing Practice: an expanded scope of practice that requires academic educational preparation in a specialty area beyond the basic nursing degree. Graduate-prepared advanced practice requires a master's degree or doctoral degree in nursing. Educational preparation for advanced practice includes a common core of knowledge in advanced practice and expanded core of knowledge in a specialty area. Preparation results in a nurse with the in-depth knowledge and skills necessary for *specialization, expansion* of knowledge and competencies, and the *advancement* of specialization and expansion which results in a new integration of theory, skills, and competencies to respond to client needs (ANA, 1996, Hickey, Ouimette, & Venegoni, 1996, pp. 1-3).

Competent Practice: practice in which care is based on planning which establishes a perspective and "Considerable conscious, abstract, analytic contemplation" (Benner, 1984/2000, p. 26) of client patterns/challenges/needs in which the nurse "lacks the speed and flexibility of the proficient nurse, but does have a feeling of mastery and the ability to cope with and manage the many contingencies of clinical nursing" (Benner, p. 27) and demonstrates efficiency and organization.

Critical Thinking: an active, purposeful, organized cognitive process involving creativity, reflection, problem solving, and both rational and intuitive judgment, attitude of inquiry, and a philosophical orientation toward thinking about thinking (adapted from many authors).

Evidence-Based Practice: the process by which nurses and other health care practitioners make clinical decisions using the best holistic nursing philosophy and theories, research evidence, clinical expertise, and patient preferences within the context of available resources.

Expert Practice: "Capturing the description of expert performance is difficult, because the expert operates from a deep understanding of the total situation..." (Benner, 1984/2000, p. 32). The expert nurse has exceptional perceptual acuity which is easily placed in context of experience an advanced clinical knowledge and skills. Expert practice demonstrates organized and networked knowledge, "a comprehensive mental library of patients, and efficient problem-solving skills" (Hickey, Ouimette, & Venegoni, 1996, p. 87).

Integrative Practice: a patient-centered and relationship-centered holistic caring process that includes the graduate-prepared holistic nurse, the client, and other health care practitioners who incorporate complementary and conventional health care services and interventions.

Proficient Practice: clinical situations are understood as a whole. Maxims are used as a guide for practice, but deep understanding of the situations is present before maxims are applied as guides rather than as absolute prescriptions. Subtle nuances of situations are understood. Recognition of significant changes in clinical situations frequently occurs prior to changes in objective data (Benner, 1984/2000, pp. 27-31).

Standards of Advanced Practice: a group of statements describing the expected level of care given by the graduate-prepared holistic nurse.

*Definitions for *AHNA Standards of Advanced Holistic Nursing Practice for Graduate-Prepared Nurses* are to be used in conjunction with the definitions provided in the *AHNA Standards of Holistic Nursing Practice.* These definitions are provided in Appendix A.

Graduate-Prepared Holistic Nursing Description

Graduate preparation in holistic nursing is aimed at specialization in a holistic approach to care. It expands the scope of holistic nursing practice through educational preparation that emphasizes critical thinking based on advanced assessment skills, advanced knowledge of physiology including psychoneuroimmunology, psychology, pharmacology, an in-depth understanding of health care policy, financing, and organization as well as advanced clinical and ethical decision-making based on holistic philosophy, theory and a broad understanding of human diversity and complex social issues and health promotion and disease prevention. Graduate preparation for the holistic nurse emphasizes a holistic perspective and expert enactment of the roles of advanced practice including clinician and facilitator of healing, consultant and collaborator, educator and guide, administrator, leader, change agent, researcher and advocate. Graduate preparation may occur at the master's and/or doctoral level.

Graduate-prepared holistic nurses (GPHNs) facilitate the healing process by using themselves as instruments of healing through the integration of advanced holistic nursing knowledge and core values of holistic nursing. GPHNs advance specialization and expansion of knowledge by influencing policymaking and holistic nursing research development and utilization. Graduate-prepared holistic nurses foster leadership in the development of the nursing profession through integration of nursing philosophy and theories, professional writing and by acting as entrepreneurs in developing models of holistic nursing practice congruent with the *AHNA Standards of Advanced Holistic Practice for Graduate-Prepared Nurses*.

Graduate-prepared holistic nurses model a wellness lifestyle, and value lifelong learning, all ways of knowing, and interconnectedness. They are aware of their assets and limitations and their effect on others and work to contribute to the well-being of individuals, families, groups, communities, and the earth. Graduate-prepared holistic nurses recognize that human beings experience reality physically, psychosocially, culturally, intellectually, and spiritually. They recognize themselves as integral to a larger universe of consciousness and endeavor to contribute in a positive and meaningful way to the larger reality.

Interventions used by graduate-prepared holistic nurses in addition to conventional nursing interventions include the interventions identified as most commonly used in holistic nursing practice (Dossey, B., Frisch, N. Forker, J. & Lavin, J., 1998) and cited in the *AHNA Standards of Holistic Nursing Practice* (AHNA, 2000) (see Appendix B) as well as the following:

- Advanced integrated assessment.
- Prescription in accordance with laws of the state in which they practice.
- Graduate-prepared holistic nurses are expected to use these interventions at the level of expert through the use of advanced knowledge of physiology including psychoneuroimmunology, holistic nursing philosophy, theory, research, and refined critical thinking skills in the use of any and all interventions.

Summary of AHNA Core Values

CORE VALUE 1: Holistic Philosophy, Theories, and Ethics
Holistic nursing practice is based on the philosophy and theory of holism and the foundation of ethical practice.

1.1   **Holistic Philosophy.** Holistic nurses develop and expand their conceptual framework and overall philosophy in the art and science of holistic nursing to effectively model, practice, teach, and conduct research.

1.2   **Holistic Theories.** Nursing theories that are holistic, and other relevant theories, provide the framework for all aspects of holistic nursing practice and leadership.

1.3   **Holistic Ethics.** Holistic nurses hold to a professional ethic of caring and healing that seeks to preserve wholeness and dignity of themselves and all persons/families/communities in all practice settings.

CORE VALUE 2: Holistic Education and Research
Holistic nursing practice is guided by, and developed through, holistic education and research.

2.1   **Holistic Education**. Holistic nurses acquire and maintain current knowledge and competency in holistic nursing practice.

2.2   **Holistic Research.** Holistic nurses provide care and guidance to persons through nursing interventions and holistic therapies consistent with research findings and other sound evidence.

CORE VALUE 3: Holistic Nurse Self-Care
Holistic nursing practice requires the integration of self-care and personal development activities into one's life.

3.1   **Holistic Nurse Self-Care**. Holistic nurses engage in holistic self-assessment, self-care, and personal development, aware of being instruments of healing to better serve self and others.

CORE VALUE 4: Holistic Communication, Therapeutic Environment, and Cultural Diversity
Holistic nursing practice honors and includes holistic communication, therapeutic environment, and cultural diversity as foundational concepts.

4.1   **Holistic Communication**. Holistic nurses engage in holistic communication to ensure that each person experiences the presence of the nurse as authentic and sincere; there is an atmosphere of shared humanness that includes a sense of connectedness and attention reflecting the individual's uniqueness.

4.2   **Therapeutic Environment.** Holistic nurses recognize that each person's environment includes everything within and surrounding the individual, as well as patterns not yet understood.

4.3   **Cultural Diversity.** Holistic nurses recognize each person as a whole body-mind-emotion-spirit being and mutually create a plan of care consistent with cultural background, health beliefs and practices, sexual orientation, values, and preferences.

CORE VALUE 5: Holistic Caring Process
Holistic nursing practice is guided by the holistic caring process, whether used with individuals, families, population groups, or communities. This circular process involves the following six steps, which may occur simultaneously.

5.1   **Assessment**. Holistic nurses assess each person holistically using appropriate conventional and holistic methods while the uniqueness of the person is honored.

5.2   **Patterns/Challenges/Needs**. Holistic nurses identify and prioritize each person's actual and potential patterns/challenges/needs and life processes related to health, wellness, disease, or illness, which may or may not facilitate well being.

5.3   **Outcomes.** Holistic nurses specify appropriate outcomes for each person's actual or potential patterns/challenges/needs.

5.4   **Therapeutic Care Plans.** Holistic nurses engage each person to mutually create an appropriate plan of care that focuses on health promotion, recovery, restoration, or peaceful dying so that the person is as independent as possible.

5.5   **Implementation**. Holistic nurses prioritize each person's plan of holistic care, and holistic nursing interventions are implemented accordingly.

5.6   **Evaluation**. Holistic nurses evaluate each person's response to holistic care regularly and systematically and the continuing holistic nature of the healing process is recognized and honored.

     Holistic Nursing: Scope and Standards of Practice

CORE VALUE 1: Holistic Philosophy, Theories, and Ethics

Holistic nursing practice is based on the philosophy and theory of holism and the foundation of ethical practice.

1.1 Holistic Philosophy
Holistic nurses develop and expand their conceptual framework and overall philosophy in the art and science of holistic nursing to effectively model, practice, teach, and conduct research.

Standards of Practice

1.1.1   Graduate-prepared holistic nurses articulate the conceptual and historical foundations of holistic nursing philosophy.

        Graduate-prepared holistic nurses articulate the ideas influencing holistic nursing philosophy, place these ideas in an historical, philosophical, and scientific context, and project future trends in thinking. Holistic philosophies are part of the history of ideas that provide a philosophical and theoretical basis for graduate holistic nursing practice. Furthermore, these ideas are not static but continually evolving. This standard recognizes the need for graduate-prepared holistic nurses to be knowledgeable about the history of ideas from which holistic nursing philosophy has developed.

1.1.2   Graduate-prepared holistic nurses express, contribute to, and promote an understanding of the following: a philosophy of nursing that values healing as the desired outcome of advanced practice caring; the human health experience as a complex, dynamic relationship of health, illness, disease and wellness; the scientific foundations of nursing practice; and nursing as an art.

        Graduate-prepared holistic nurses are often called to teach, present, and lead others in developing care models and providing care. They apply holistic philosophy to practice and provide guidance to others in this process. They contribute to developing holistic philosophies that integrate the humanities and sciences including nursing science and the scientific tradition of biomedicine.

1.1.3   Graduate-prepared holistic nurses believe that it is necessary to understand the client's health experience from the client's perspective.

        Graduate-prepared holistic nurses emphasize a philosophy that recognizes clients as the authority on their own health experience and encourages an ethic that values this experience. It recognizes that context is necessary to understanding the health experience. Therefore, graduate-prepared holistic nurses elicit and use client narratives to guide care whenever possible. These narratives, whether they arise from individuals, families, groups or communities, reveal the context and complexity of the health experience.

1.1.4   Graduate-prepared holistic nurses believe that holistic care arises from a context of care that is relationship-centered, scientific, aesthetic, culturally and socially sensitive, and ecologically sound.

        Graduate-prepared holistic nurses create practice environments with clients and with other professionals. They philosophically support the development of practices that are relationship-centered, scientific, artful, attentive to complex contextual factors, and that sustain the environment. Furthermore, graduate-prepared holistic nurses teach and influence other nurses toward this kind of practice. They promote holistic philosophy in the workplace, contribute to the body of scholarly knowledge deriving from holistic philosophy, and promote interdisciplinary understanding of holistic philosophy.

1.2 Holistic Theories
Nursing theories that are holistic, and other relevant theories, provide the framework for all aspects of holistic nursing practice and leadership.

Standards of Practice

1.2.1   Graduate-prepared holistic nurses identify, critique, modify, adapt, and evaluate theories that have relevance for nursing.

Graduate-prepared holistic nurses examine theories from many disciplines to implement this standard. Therefore, they demonstrate interdisciplinary knowledge. They are especially attentive to theories from other disciplines that might contribute to holistic nursing practice. They understand the metaparadigm of nursing and its relationship to holistic thinking. They can describe the essential elements of a holistic nursing theory and evaluate existing and emerging nursing theories for application to holistic nursing practice. Graduate-prepared holistic nurses understanding the process of theory development, the various types of theories, and the relationship of theory to practice and research.

1.2.2   Graduate-prepared holistic nurses use relevant theories from nursing and other disciplines in their advanced practice.

Graduate-prepared holistic nurses create their practices from a sound theoretical basis that expresses holistic philosophy and ethics, holistic care relationships, and holistic interventions. Graduate-prepared holistic nurses use holistic theories rather than comprehensive theories to establish and guide their practice (see definitions). They interpret, use and document information relevant to advanced practice using a theoretical framework.

1.2.3   Graduate-prepared holistic nurses participate in theory development in nursing. Graduate-prepared holistic nurses generate and test theories and contribute to scholarly discourse on current theories.

1.3 Holistic Ethics
Holistic nurses hold to a professional ethic of caring and healing that seeks to preserve wholeness and dignity of themselves and all persons/families/communities in all practice settings.

Standards of Practice

1.3.1   Graduate-prepared holistic nurses articulate the ethical foundations of advanced holistic practice.

Graduate-prepared holistic nurses recognize the values and ethics of holistic care that are grounded in a history of ethical thought. Graduate-prepared holistic nurses explore these ethical foundations, including major concepts, values, approaches to decision-making and the ethical issues in nursing research. Graduate-prepared holistic nurses articulate and value nursing ethics and the ethic of care and the tradition of biomedical (principle-oriented) ethics. They analyze and synthesize ethical traditions to develop moral insight and decision-making skills. They influence others toward a holistic perspective of ethical situations and decisions making.

1.3.2   Graduate-prepared holistic nurses value and demonstrate the *American Holistic Nurses Association Code of Ethics* in their advanced practice.

Graduate-prepared holistic nurses integrate the *AHNA Code of Ethics* to help articulate the moral foundation of holistic nursing. It is appropriate for all levels of holistic nursing practice. However, the graduate-prepared nurse discusses this Code with others, and creates a practice that honors this Code regardless of setting and complexity of client situations. Furthermore, they participate in revisions of the Code as deemed necessary by the organization. Graduate-prepared nurses conduct research that embodies the values of the *AHNA Code of Ethics*. They identify areas of personal conflict, clarify personal values, and demonstrate integrity in all the roles of the advanced practice nurse. Integrity means taking time to deliberate about one's moral position, acting in accordance with that position and being accountable for the outcomes of decisions made based on that position (Carter, 1996). They understand the role of ethics committees and may create and participate on them.

1.3.3   Graduate-prepared holistic nurses integrate these standards for advanced holistic practice with the laws, rules, and regulations that govern advanced practice nursing.

Graduate-prepared nurses are familiar with the laws, rules, and regulations in their state that govern their practice. Their practices reflect an understanding of the legal basis for practice as well as the ethical dimensions of various practice settings. They develop practice protocols and provide therapies and interventions within legal parameters. They may also work within the legal system to challenge current laws and regulations using research (qualitative and quantitative) as a basis for change affecting the well-being of clients and society. Graduate-prepared holistic nurses may use organized political action and advocacy to change unresponsive systems.

1.3.4   Graduate-prepared holistic nurses are responsible and accountable for their advanced practice.

Graduate-prepared holistic nurses take full legal and ethical accountability for their practice. They maintain necessary licenses and certifications and practice within the laws, rules and regulations for advanced nursing practice. They know and practice using applicable standards that include but are not limited to the *AHNA Standards of Advanced Holistic Practice Nursing for Graduate-Prepared Nurses*. They document care thoroughly and appropriately. They make ethical decisions congruent with their personal code of ethics, the *AHNA Code of Ethics*, and other applicable Codes.

1.3.5   Graduate-prepared holistic nurses are advocates for the rights of vulnerable populations.

Graduate-prepared holistic nurses enact the advanced practice role of advocate based on the increased level of responsibility and accountability of graduate preparation. They support human dignity through advocacy and adherence to the *Patient's Bill of Rights*. Holistic ethics and the moral foundation of nursing dictate that the graduate-prepared holistic nurse act on behalf of clients including families groups, and communities who cannot seek or demand ethical treatment on their own. Advanced practice graduate-prepared holistic nurses may also act as advocates for other nurses and colleagues.

CORE VALUE 2: Holistic Education and Research

Holistic nursing practice is guided by, and developed through, holistic education and research.

2.1 Holistic Education
Holistic nurses acquire and maintain current knowledge and competency in holistic nursing practice.

Standards of Practice

2.1.1   Graduate-prepared holistic nurses hold a graduate degree demonstrating coursework and supervised clinical practice that reflects the *American Holistic Nurses Association Standards of Advanced Holistic Practice for Graduate-Prepared Nurses.*

The entry level for advanced practice is a graduate degree. Four specializations have been recognized by the American Nurses Association as a basis for advanced practice requiring education and or certification beyond the basic level. These are the Clinical Nurse Specialist (CNS), nurse practitioner (NP), nurse anesthetist (CRNA), and nurse midwife (CNM) (ANA, 1996). This standard recognizes that graduate nursing programs to prepare nurses for advanced holistic practice are emerging. The intent of this standard is to provide a guide for graduate curriculum design emphasizing a holistic perspective. It is recognized and valued that many graduate-prepared nurses have created a holistic basis for their work as clinicians, administrators, or educators through interdisciplinary study and degrees, continuing education, or by selecting learning opportunities in more traditional nursing programs for study from a holistic perspective.

2.1.2   Graduate-prepared holistic nurses engage in lifelong learning.

Graduate-prepared holistic nurses demonstrate commitment to life long learning in a variety of ways including but not limited to holistic nurse certification, continuing education, other certifications, and additional degree seeking programs. Furthermore, graduate-prepared holistic nurses stay current with nursing literature, including journals, books, and Internet offerings. They also contribute to the literature and provide continuing education for others. They are aware of changes in national standards for practice and trends in nursing education.

2.1.3   Graduate-prepared holistic nurses educate others in ways that demonstrate a holistic philosophy and ethic that value all ways of knowing and learning.

Graduate-prepared holistic nurses as educators develop a philosophy of teaching and learning that is holistic. They educate others based on this philosophy and create educational environments that are safe for the exploration necessary to learning. They determine readiness and motivation for learning and for maintaining health-related activities using principles of change theory. The need for client teaching is based on anticipatory guidance associated with growth and development, care management that requires specific information and skills, and the client need for further understanding of the health experience. Graduate-prepared holistic nurses elicit information about perceived barriers, supports, and modifiers to learning as part of the routine health assessment. They use discretionary judgment in assessing conflicting teaching/learning priorities and needs. They assist others to access inner wisdom that can provide opportunities to enhance and support growth, development and wholeness.

2.2 Holistic Research
Holistic nurses provide care and guidance to persons through nursing interventions and holistic therapies consistent with research findings and other sound evidence.

Standards of Practice

2.2.1   Graduate-prepared holistic nurses are proficient in analyzing and evaluating research studies.

Graduate-prepared holistic nurses have advanced knowledge and skill to critically analyze the conception, design, and analysis and reporting of the findings of both qualitative and quantitative research studies.

2.2.2   Graduate-prepared holistic nurses use research as a basis for developing the roles of the advanced practice, making care decisions with individuals, families, groups and communities, and engaging in self-care and care of the environment.

Graduate-prepared holistic nurses develop evidenced-based advanced practices relying on the best research available, current practice guidelines, clinical expertise, and client values. They make necessary changes in practice in accord with the best available evidence.

2.2.3   Graduate-prepared holistic nurses participate in and conduct research that is rigorous in scholarship, philosophically congruent, and that demonstrates ethical integrity while contributing to the body of nursing knowledge.

Graduate-prepared holistic nurses with research experience conduct both qualitative and quantitative research studies. These studies investigate questions or phenomena of particular concern to advanced holistic nursing practice. They demonstrate a holistic philosophical basis and are ethically sound.

2.2.4   Graduate-prepared holistic nurses participate with others to identify research questions or areas for inquiry and set research priorities.

Graduate-prepared holistic nurses participate in the development of research agendas in professional organizations and in the workplace. They identify potential research questions that nurses consider of high clinical significance in improving the quality of patient care. They prioritize research questions using criteria to determine clinical significance. They select research questions to be investigated and create research opportunities. Research questions that have the potential to add to the philosophical, theoretical, ethical or contextual aspect of holistic nursing are also identified and pursued.

2.2.5   Graduate-prepared holistic nurses consult with others when needed to design studies, analyze data, interpret results, and report findings.

Graduate-prepared holistic nurses consult with others in conducting clinical research when additional expertise is required. They may consult with mentors when identifying research problems and funding opportunities, initiating proposal writing, seeking institutional approval to protect the rights of human subjects in research, facilitating implementation and maintenance of study data collection, preparing raw data for computer analysis, interpreting study results, and in preparing the final research report.

2.2.6   Graduate-prepared holistic nurses communicate research results in both professional and general-audience publications and presentations.

Graduate-prepared holistic nurses present research results and the implications of the findings for holistic nursing practice at appropriate local, regional, national, and international professional meetings. They publish research results, implications for clinical practice, and recommendations for future research in appropriate peer-reviewed journals. They are able to interpret research results for a wide variety of audiences including the public and other disciplines.

2.2.7   Graduate-prepared holistic nurses participate in interdisciplinary discourse and research.

Graduate-prepared holistic nurses represent the voice of holistic nursing in interdisciplinary discourse about clinical research. They discuss ways to evaluate the integration of body-mind-spirit therapies to achieve optimal patient outcomes. They help to facilitate the holistic and ethical focus of clinical problems in a way that furthers group cohesion. They serve as principle investigators, co-investigators, and research coordinators for interdisciplinary research studies.

2.2.8   Graduate-prepared holistic nurses use quality improvement methods, research, and program evaluation to evaluate holistic outcomes for individuals, population groups, and communities.

Graduate-prepared holistic nurses use quality improvement techniques and skills to monitor and improve practice. Quality care activities include developing quality indicators, measuring care against standards and analyzing data. Quality care activities may also include program evaluations and qualitative research to determine quality of care. Graduate-prepared holistic nurses design quality care programs and evaluate both qualitative and quantitative data. Program decisions are based on data generated by quality improvement activities.

CORE VALUE 3: Holistic Nurse Self-Care

Holistic nursing practice requires the integration of self-care and personal development activities into one's life.

3.1 Holistic Nurse Self-Care
Holistic nurses engage in holistic self-assessment, self-care, and personal development, aware of being instruments of healing to better serve self and others.

Standards of Practice

3.1.1   Graduate-prepared holistic nurses value themselves and their calling to advanced holistic nursing practice as a life purpose.

Graduate-prepared holistic nurses value themselves; and enlist the necessary resources to care for themselves. They recognize the uniqueness and complexity of the interaction of the physical body, the psychological-social-cultural self, the intellectual self, and the spiritual self. However, they do not equate physical health with spiritual health or confuse manifestations of suffering, discomfort, injury, or disease with inadequacy, but rather with the need for attention and learning that come with these experiences which are a natural part of the human health experience. They are concerned with fulfilling a life purpose that has its focus in service to others while not neglecting their own well-being. The increased accountability and greater responsibilities of advanced practice creates increased requirements for attention to self-care.

3.1.2   Graduate-prepared holistic nurses design, implement, and evaluate their self-care recognizing their uniqueness and the rhythms and cycles of life.

Graduate-prepared holistic nurses are the experts on their own health experience. They reflect on their health experience to discover life patterns of self-care practices and responses. They realize that advanced practice changes the level of commitment to nursing and changes the patterns of life to work. They recognize and attend to the necessary changes in relationships that the increased accountability, commitment and responsibility of advanced practice bring. They are knowledgeable about various approaches to self-assessment and complementary and alternative health practices. They integrate self-care into their lives and engage in self-management in ways that honor their unique patterns and the cycles of growth and development of the body, the psychological-social-cultural self, the intellectual self, and the spiritual self.

3.1.3   Graduate-prepared holistic nurses value all life experiences as opportunities to find meaning and cultivate self-awareness, self-reflection, and growth.

Graduate-prepared holistic nurses understand that finding meaning in experience is healing. They know that suffering is as much a part of life as joy and that all experiences have the potential to teach us about our Universe and ourselves. Thus, they value every experience and the unique structure and patterns of their own lives, the lives of others, of nature and the Universe. Through reflective practice they recognize their assets and limitations. They acknowledge that change is difficult and seek appropriate resources when needed for their own well-being.

3.1.4   Graduate-prepared holistic nurses honor their creative selves through aesthetic self-expression.

Graduate-prepared holistic nurses use creative expression as a way of knowing that helps to find meaning in life experience. They are all creative and creative expression is demonstrated in many ways. Some of these ways are through traditional art forms, but creativity is also expressed in originality and innovation in practice, teaching, management or research. This standard asks the advanced practice nurse to honor the creative self by recognizing it and giving it expression in a way that adds beauty to their lives and their practice. Giving expression to personal creativity enables the advanced practice nurse to assist their clients more creatively and to honor the creative process of their clients.

CORE VALUE 4: Holistic Communication, Therapeutic Environment, and Cultural Diversity

Holistic nursing practice honors and includes holistic communication, therapeutic environment, and cultural diversity as foundational concepts.

4.1 Holistic Communication
Holistic nurses engage in holistic communication to ensure that each person experiences the presence of the nurse as authentic and sincere; there is an atmosphere of shared humanness that includes a sense of connectedness and attention reflecting the individual's uniqueness.

Standards of Practice

4.1.1   Graduate-prepared holistic nurses establish practice environments that recognize and value holistic communication as fundamental to holistic care.

Graduate-prepared holistic nurses have the responsibility for creating with others the communication atmosphere of the practice environment. How they communicate is a significant factor in their effectiveness as advanced practitioners. Therefore, advanced practice graduate-prepared holistic nurses recognize that communication, verbal and nonverbal, linguistic and symbolic, is a visible expression of the art of nursing. They endeavor to communicate artfully, clearly, accurately, and sensitively with everyone in the practice environment. They validate their interpretations of what has been communicated and acknowledge the importance of context in understanding the health experience. They engage with others in a way that demonstrates an altruistic impulse toward others and a willingness to extend oneself while maintaining appropriate psychological boundaries.

4.1.2   Graduate-prepared holistic nurses express mutuality in their communication with others.

Graduate-prepared holistic nurses establish practice settings that promote mutuality while honoring the psychological boundaries of themselves and others. Mutuality demonstrates interconnectedness and empathy in the sense of feeling oneself into another's experience. In mutuality the advanced practice nurse is authentically and fully present to others.

4.1.3   Graduate-prepared holistic nurses use linguistic and symbolic language to explore with their clients the potentials, possibilities, innovations, options, and meaning in the health experience.

Graduate-prepared holistic nurses communicate for the purpose of exploration which allows for open, intuitive, metaphoric, and heuristic ways of expression. They are comfortable with ambiguity, paradox, uncertainty, and unknowing. When the nurse accepts unknowing as a necessary aspect of holistic communication, a sacred space is created for both nurse and client to explore. Graduate-prepared holistic nurses establish practice settings that allow others the space and time for exploration. They support others during the confusion and doubt that are a necessary part of exploration. Exploration underscores the fact that each health experience is unique and may be at odds with current knowledge.

4.1.4 Graduate-prepared holistic nurses recognize and honor the unique rhythms and patterns of relating that are expressed in communication.

Graduate-prepared holistic nurses recognize that each relationship has a unique rhythm and pattern of relating. The dynamics of relating reveal themselves in rhythm (the going back and forth of communication, such as listening-talking, touching-not touching, hope-hopelessness, certainty-uncertainty) and in the movement through the holistic nursing relationship from beginning to end. They create practice settings that support these unique rhythms and patterns. They have a heightened sensitivity to these rhythms and patterns and a sense of timing that is intuitive and that honors this uniqueness.

4.1.5 Graduate-prepared holistic nurses recognize and explore the meanings of the symbolic language that are a part of the individual's health experience.

Graduate-prepared holistic nurses have an expanded knowledge base in the use and meanings of symbolic language. Symbolic language, such as that found in dreams, cultural myths and rituals including prayer and meditation, imagery and art is an integral aspect of the health experience. With adequate educational preparation, graduate-prepared holistic nurses incorporate in their practices therapies based on symbolic language such as imagery, creation of sacred space and personal rituals, dream exploration, and the use of aesthetic therapies such as music, visual art, and dance. Graduate-prepared holistic nurses encourage and support others in the use of prayer, meditation or other spiritual and symbolic practices for healing purposes.

4.2. Therapeutic Environment
Holistic nurses recognize that each person's environment includes everything within and surrounding the individual, as well as patterns not yet understood.

Standards of Practice

4.2.1 Graduate-prepared holistic nurses create integrative practice environments conducive to healing.

Graduate-prepared holistic nurses collaborate and consult with others to provide care for individuals, families, groups, and communities that integrate conventional biomedical, complementary, and alternative approaches to healing. Care is not limited to disease treatment, but includes health promotion, health restoration and disease prevention.

4.2.2 Graduate-prepared holistic nurses lead organizations in creating therapeutic environments that value holistic caring, social support, and healing.

Graduate-prepared holistic nurses are leaders and change agents who work to create organizations that accept, support, and promote the use of integrated approaches to care that is safe, efficacious, and cost effective. Further, as leaders, graduate-prepared holistic nurses are in a unique position to acknowledge the contributions and practices of other nurses. They offer peer support, consultation and mentoring of others. They identify and help to create social networks and environments in which individuals feel connected, supported, and valued.

4.2.3 Graduate-prepared holistic nurses create policies, procedures, and standards in care settings that integrate holistic philosophy and principles with environmental safety and emergency preparedness.

Graduate-prepared holistic nurses act as leaders, collaborators, consultants, and change agents in evaluating environmental safety, anticipating the potential effect of environmental hazards on the health or welfare of individuals, groups and communities, and assisting in reducing or eliminating environmental hazards. They use community assessment information and apply principles of epidemiology in clinical practice. They recognize the impact of life threatening factors for people associated with emergencies such as earthquakes, tornadoes and hurricanes, and man-made disasters and promote the integration of a holistic perspective with nationally accepted guidelines and standards for emergency preparedness.

4.2.4   Graduate-prepared holistic nurses actively contribute to creating an ecosystem that supports well-being for all life.

Graduate-prepared holistic nurses recognize the impact of global health care issues on individuals, groups, communities and all living things. They engage in activities to promote solutions to health problems that are mutually beneficial to all involved. Graduate-prepared holistic nurses use practical ways to cope with hazards or consequences of environmental stressors. They conduct research and apply research findings that link environmental hazards and human response patterns. They promote choices for a healthy environment, safety in the workplace, and engage in consciousness-raising about environmental issues. They respond when international laws or global environmental issues contribute to the transmission of public health disease. They are advocates for social justice and the rights of the repressed.

4.2.5   Graduate-prepared holistic nurses are knowledgeable about the organization, policies, and financing of the health care system.

Graduate-prepared holistic nurses articulate how health care is organized, delivered, and financed for individuals, population groups, and communities. They understand the political barriers to holistic care and work to eliminate these barriers and provide leadership in health care delivery in a variety of settings through the diverse roles of the advanced practice nurse. They have an expanded knowledge base of organizational dynamics and processes of organizational change.

4.3 Cultural Diversity
Holistic nurses recognize each person as a whole body-mind-emotion-spirit being and mutually create a plan of care consistent with cultural background, health beliefs and practices, sexual orientation, values, and preferences.

Standards of Practice

4.3.1   Graduate-prepared holistic nurses create practice environments that are non-discriminatory and culturally and socially competent.

Graduate-prepared holistic nurses have a global perspective of health care problems that result from social issues and lifestyle choices. They create practice environments for clients that are non-discriminatory and that do not suppress their many diverse beliefs about the etiology of disease and the many possible approaches to healing. Further, through expanded knowledge about culturally sensitive care, graduate-prepared nurses demonstrate moral insight related to client rights to care. They seek to eliminate artificial barriers such as affordability and accessibility which create added risks for persons of varied racial, ethnic, and social backgrounds. They implement policies to prevent discrimination.

4.3.2   Graduate-prepared holistic nurses provide care with individual clients, families, groups, and communities that is non-discriminatory and culturally and socially congruent.

Graduate-prepared holistic nurses reflect on their own cultural beliefs, practices, and values and assess the impact of these on their ability to provide culturally and socially sensitive care. They possess the knowledge and understanding of a wide range of cultural norms and health care practices concerning individuals, families, groups and communities from varied racial, ethnic, and social backgrounds. They use this expanded knowledge base to provide care that is culturally and socially competent and congruent with the beliefs, values, and practices of clients.

4.3.3   Graduate-prepared holistic nurses provide leadership and mentorship of others in providing non-discriminatory, socially and culturally congruent care.

Graduate-prepared holistic nurses provide leadership and mentor others by serving as exemplars modeling specific values and professional behaviors that can be emulated. For example, teaching specific skills that are considered to be complementary and alternative in one culture, yet, mainstream in another are professional competencies in holistic practice that are performed in a non-discriminatory and socially congruent manner. Successfully mentoring one to achieve professional growth is a positive and fulfilling experience that leads to satisfaction for the protégé, the mentor, and the profession.

4.3.4 Graduate-prepared holistic nurses are leaders in establishing resources to provide non-discriminatory, socially and culturally congruent care.

Graduate-prepared holistic nurses make referrals to services that provide culturally and socially congruent non-discriminatory care. They assist clients to organize and integrate resources of other agencies or care providers to meet client needs and assist in problem resolution.

CORE VALUE 5: Holistic Caring Process

Holistic nursing practice is guided by the holistic caring process, whether used with individuals, families, population groups, or communities. This circular process involves the following six steps, which may occur simultaneously.

5.1 Assessment
Holistic nurses assess each person holistically using appropriate conventional and holistic methods while the uniqueness of the person is honored.

Standards of Practice

5.1.1 Graduate-prepared holistic nurses conduct advanced holistic assessments based on theory, current research findings, and evolving self/intuitive knowing.

Graduate-prepared holistic nurses conduct advanced holistic assessment that is thorough and includes developing a holistic database demonstrating equal proficiency in physical, functional, psychosocial, emotional, mental, cultural, spiritual, transpersonal and energy field assessments across the lifespan, and analysis and synthesize data as they relate to the whole person within the life context. Assessment includes principles of epidemiology and demography as part of the assessment process. Both medical and nursing diagnoses are used in assessment findings.

Graduate-prepared holistic nurses use appropriate laboratory and other diagnostic tests as indicated for accurate and thorough assessment. When assessing client groups or communities, the graduate-prepared holistic nurse considers all the realms of human existence: physical, functional, psychosocial, emotional, cultural, mental, and spiritual/transpersonal aspects of the group and demonstrates knowledge of group and community dynamics that may include consideration of group energy field dynamics and patterns.

5.2 Patterns/Challenges/Needs
Holistic nurses identify and prioritize each person's actual and potential patterns/challenges/needs and life processes related to health, wellness, disease, or illness, which may or may not facilitate well being.

Standards of Practice

5.2.1 Graduate-prepared holistic nurses translate assessment data as patterns/challenges/needs from which meaning and understanding of the health/disease experience can be mutually identified with the client.

Graduate-prepared holistic nurses demonstrate critical thinking and diagnostic-reasoning skills in clinical decision-making. Based on advanced knowledge of physiology, pathophysiology, and psychology, differential diagnoses are established. Appropriate laboratory, common screening and/or other diagnostic tests are prescribed and interpreted as indicated. Graduate-prepared holistic nurses use assessment findings (including medical and nursing) in creating a holistic diagnosis. They diagnose the level of acuity, severity, and complexity of health patterns/challenges/needs and appropriately consult, collaborate, prescribe, and refer to both conventional medical providers as well as other holistic providers. They assist the client in recognizing at-risk patterns/challenges/needs for potential or existing health situations (e.g., lifestyle/personal habits, personal and family health history, age-related risk factors), and also assist in recognizing opportunities to enhance well-being.

5.3 Outcomes
Holistic nurses specify appropriate outcomes for each person's actual or potential patterns/challenges/needs.

Standards of Practice

5.3.1   Graduate-prepared holistic nurses anticipate and mutually formulate the client health experience outcomes based ient understanding and meanings in their patterns and processes.

Graduate-prepared holistic nurses identify with clients expected quantitative/qualitative outcomes in consideration of the associated risks, benefits, and costs of care. They value the evolution of spirit and the process of healing as it unfolds. This implies that specific unfolding outcomes may not be evident immediately due to the nonlinear nature of the healing process.

5.4 Therapeutic Care Plans
Holistic nurses engage each person to mutually create an appropriate plan of care that focuses on health promotion, recovery, restoration, or peaceful dying so that the person is as independent as possible.

Standards of Practice

5.4.1   Graduate-prepared holistic nurses mutually create dynamic plans of care that respect the client's health experience while promoting choice and individuation, and include strategies for health, wholeness, and growth along the lifespan continuum.

Graduate-prepared holistic nurses use skills of cultural competence and communicate acceptance of the client's values, beliefs, culture, religion and socioeconomic background and provide clients with information that is scientifically grounded and appropriate to the health condition including a description of what the condition is, proposed therapies, therapeutic effects, and side effects.

5.5 Implementation
Holistic nurses prioritize each person's plan of holistic care, and holistic nursing interventions are implemented accordingly.

Standards of Practice

5.5.1   Graduate-prepared holistic nurses implement care within the scope of practice of advanced practice registered nursing and in accordance with State and Federal laws and regulations.

Graduate-prepared holistic nurses implement culturally competent and ethical care based on the outcomes of advanced holistic assessment. They honor client plans, choices, boundaries, and the uniqueness of each healing journey. They employ therapeutic research/theory-based interventions with attention to safety, invasiveness, simplicity, acceptability, and efficacy. They provide guidance and counseling to clients in all aspects of the health experience and throughout the lifespan. They provide information and counseling regarding holistic/complementary/integrative and conventional health care services and guide clients and families. Graduate-prepared holistic nurses prescribe medications as legally authorized and counsel clients concerning drug/herbal/homeopathic regimens as well as drug/herbal/homeopathic side effects and interactions. They facilitate the negotiation of holistic/complementary/integrative and conventional health care services and provide follow-up for continuity of care for the client and for program planning. They develop a documentation system that communicates client health status verbally or in writing using appropriate terminology and format to ensure that clients receive appropriate services. They coordinate human and environmental resources necessary to manage changing situations and assist clients in using community resources. They provide case management services to meet multiple client health care needs over time.

5.5.2   Graduate-prepared holistic nurses use advanced knowledge of pharmacology, nutritional supplements, herbal and homeopathic remedies, and a variety of complementary and alternative therapies.

Graduate-prepared holistic nurses prescribe treatment interventions according to client health care needs and based on current knowledge, practice and research. The research base regarding nutritional supplements, herbal and homeopathic remedies, and complementary and alternative treatments is expanding; however it does not yet support all treatment recommendations, some of which have a long history of efficacious use. Graduate-prepared holistic nurses accurately report to clients the research findings regarding selected treatments. When no such research results have been established, this is also reported to the client along with the history of usage. Graduate-prepared holistic nurses prescribe specific agents and/or treatments based on clinical indicators or on the client's status and needs, including the results of diagnostic and laboratory tests, as appropriate. They monitor intended effects and potential adverse effects of treatments. They provide the client with appropriate information about intended effects, potential adverse effects of the proposed prescribed agents/treatments, costs, and alternative treatments and procedures and analyze the effects of single and multiple interventions and the client's health and functioning. Graduate-prepared holistic nurses with prescriptive authority practice within the guidelines established by the state in which they are practicing.

5.5.3   Graduate-prepared holistic nurses demonstrate competency in a variety of role dimensions including expert clinician and facilitator of healing; consultant and collaborator; educator and guide; administrator, leader and change agent; researcher and advocate.

Graduate-prepared holistic nurses demonstrate, implement and use an expansion of knowledge and skills beyond the basic level and a high level of integration of theories, skills, and competencies in the various role dimensions of advanced practice. Advanced practice builds on basic practice and requires a higher level of expertise in all roles. Graduate-prepared holistic nurses have the depth and breadth of knowledge, skills, and competencies required for advanced practice role performance including the ability to analyze and synthesize complicated data, respond to complex situations, and to interpret these data and situations from a holistic perspective. They demonstrate a high degree of autonomy in decision-making and direct accountability to clients and colleagues. They contribute to interdisciplinary discourse and care. They practice with advanced knowledge and skills in a variety of health care situations and settings and wherever healing might occur. In all these capacities, they uphold a holistic philosophy. Furthermore, graduate-prepared holistic nurses interpret and market the advanced practice holistic nurse role to the public and other health care professions.

5.5.4   Graduate-prepared holistic nurses demonstrate decision-making in advanced practice by proficient use of many ways of knowing in implementing the holistic caring process.

Graduate-prepared holistic nurses accept as a premise that all behavior has meaning, purpose and can be understood. They honor the healing intent of all behavior and integrate the appreciation of the wholeness and beauty of the human condition into the decision-making process and partner with the client in decision-making. Empirical, ethical, aesthetic, personal, and sociological ways of knowing are used in decision-making.

5.6 Evaluation
Holistic nurses evaluate each person's response to holistic care regularly and systematically and the continuing holistic nature of the healing process is recognized and honored.

Standards of Practice

5.6.1   Graduate-prepared holistic nurses monitor client behaviors and specific outcomes as a useful guide to evaluating the effectiveness of interventions.

Graduate-prepared holistic nurses use formal/informal evaluation methods to determine with clients if care is holistic, appropriate, and effective. They work to understand the cause of any significant deviation between the responses and the expected outcomes. Evaluation of changes/transformations of meaning in the health experience is also considered. They mutually create with clients and other team members a revised plan if needed.

References

American Association of Colleges of Nursing. (1996). *The essentials of master's education.* Washington, D.C.: AACN.

American Holistic Nurses Association (2004). *Standards of holistic nursing practice.* Flagstaff, AZ: AHNA.

American Nurses Association (1996). *Scope and standards of advanced practice registered nursing.* Washington, D.C.: ANA.

Benner, P. (1984/2000). *From novice to expert: Excellence and power in clinical nursing practice. Commemorative Edition.* New Jersey: Prentice-Hall.

Carter, S.J. (1996). *Integrity.* New York: HarperPerennial.

Frisch, N.C., Dossey, B.M., Guzzetta, C.E., & Quinn, J.A. (2000). *American Holistic Nurses standards of practice: Guidelines for caring and healing.* Gaithersburg, MD: Aspen.

Hickey, J. V., Ouimette, R.M., & Venegoni, S.L. (2000). *Advanced practice nursing: Changing roles and clinical applications.* (2nd ed.). Baltimore, MD: Lippincott, Williams, & Wilkins.

Additional Resources

Dossey, B.M., Keegan, L., and Guzzetta, C.E. (2004). *Holistic nursing: A handbook for practice.* (4th ed.) Gaithersburg, MD: Aspen.

Dossey, B.M. (Editor) (1997). *American Holistic Nurses Association core curriculum for holistic nursing.* Gaithersburg, MD: Aspen.

Appendix A
AHNA Holistic Nursing Practice Definitions
(From the AHNA Standards of Holistic Nursing Practice)

Allopathic/Traditional Therapies: medical, surgery, invasive and noninvasive diagnostic treatment procedures, including medications.

Caring-Healing Interventions: nontraditional therapies that can interface with traditional medical and surgical therapies; may be used as complements to conventional medical and surgical treatments; also called alternative/complementary/integrative therapies or interventions. See list of interventions most frequently used in holistic nursing practice (Appendix B).

Client of Holistic Nursing: an individual, family, group, or community of persons who is engaged in interactions with a holistic nurse in a manner respectful of each client's subjective experience about health, health beliefs, values, sexual orientation, and personal preferences.

Cultural Competence: the ability to deliver health care with knowledge of and sensitivity to cultural factors that influence the health behavior of the person.

Environment: everything that surrounds the person, both the external and the internal (physical, mental, emotional, social, and spiritual) environment as well as patterns not yet understood.

Healing: the process of bringing together aspects of one's self, body-mind-spirit, at deeper levels of inner knowing leading toward integration and balance with each aspect having equal importance and value; can lead to more complex levels of personal understanding and meaning; may be synchronous but not synonymous with curing.

Healing Process: a continual journey of changing and evolving of one's self through life; the awareness of patterns that support or are challenges/barriers to health and healing; may be done alone or in a healing community.

Health: the state or process in which the individual (nurse, client, family, group, or community) experiences a sense of well-being, harmony, and unity where subjective experiences about health, health beliefs, and values are honored.

Health Promotion: activities and preventive measures such as immunizations, fitness/exercise programs, breast self exam, appropriate nutrition, relaxation, stress management, social support, prayer, meditation, healing rituals, cultural practices, and promoting environmental health and safety.

Holistic Caring Process: a circular process that involves six steps which may occur simultaneously. These parts are assessment, patterns/challenges/needs, outcomes, therapeutic care plan, implementation, and evaluation.

Holistic Communication: a free flow of verbal and nonverbal interchange between and among people and significant beings such as pets, nature, and God/Life Force/Absolute/Transcendent that explores meaning and ideas leading to mutual understanding and growth.

Holistic Nurse: a nurse who recognizes and integrates body-mind-spirit principles and modalities in daily life and clinical practice; one who creates a healing space within herself/himself that allows the nurse to be an instrument of healing for the purpose of helping another feel safe and more in harmony; one who shares authenticity of unconditional presence that helps to remove the barriers to the healing process.

Human Caring Process: the moral state in which the holistic nurse brings her or his whole self into relationship to the whole self of significant beings which reinforces the meaning and experience of oneness and unity.

Intention: the conscious awareness of being in the present moment to help facilitate the healing process; a volitional act of love.

Intuition: perceived knowing of things and events without the conscious use of rational processes; using all the senses to receive information.

Patterns/Challenges/Needs: a person's actual and potential life processes related to health, wellness, disease, or illness which may or may not facilitate well-being.

Person: an individual, client, patient, family member, support person, or community member who has the opportunity to engage in interaction with a holistic nurse.

Person-Centered Care: the condition of trust that is created where holistic care can be given and received; the human caring process in which the holistic nurse gives full attention and intention to the whole self of a person, not merely the current presenting symptoms, illness, crisis, or tasks to be accomplished; reinforcing the person's meaning and experience of communion and unity.

Presence: the essential state or core in healing; approaching an individual in a way that respects and honors her/his essence; relating in a way that reflects a quality of *being with* and *in collaboration with* rather than *doing to; entering* into a shared experience (or field of consciousness) that promotes healing potentials and an experience of well-being.

Spirituality: a unifying force of a person; the essence of being that permeates all of life and is manifested in one's being, knowing, and doing; the interconnectedness with self, others, nature, and God/Life Force/ Absolute/ Transcendent.

Standards of Practice: a group of statements describing the expected level of care by a holistic nurse.

Interventions Most Frequently Used In Holistic Nursing Practice[1]

Acupressure

Aromatherapy

Art Therapy

Biofeedback

Cognitive Therapy

Counseling[2]

Exercise and Movement

Goal-Setting and Contracts

Guided Imagery

Healing Presence

Healing Touch Modalities

Holistic Self-Assessments

Humor and Laughter

Journaling

Massage

Meditation

Music and Sound Therapy

Nutrition Counseling

Play Therapy

Prayer

Reflexology

Relaxation Modalities

Self-Care Interventions

Self-Reflection

Smoking Cessation

Therapeutic Touch

Weight Management

---

1   See Dossey, B., Frisch, N., Forker, J., and Lavin, J. Evolving a Blueprint for Certification: Inventory of Professional Activities and Knowledge of a Holistic Nurse, *Journal of Holistic Nursing,* 1998, Vol. 16, No. 1, p 33—56.

2   Used in situations such as addictions, death and grief; unhealthy environments, relationship issues, sexual abuse, spiritual needs, violence, support groups, wellness promotion, and life-style issues.

APPENDIX D
AHNA POSITION STATEMENTS

American Holistic Nurses Association. (2007). *Position on Holistic Nursing Ethics*. Flagstaff, AZ: AHNA.

American Holistic Nurses Association. (2007). *Position on Nursing Research and Scholarship*. Flagstaff, AZ: AHNA.

American Holistic Nurses Association. (2007). *Position on the Role of Nurses in the Practice of Complementary and Alternative Therapies*. Flagstaff, AZ: AHNA.

POSITION ON HOLISTIC NURSING ETHICS

Code of Ethics for Holistic Nurses

We believe that the fundamental responsibilities of the nurse are to promote health, facilitate healing, and alleviate suffering. The need for nursing is universal. Inherent in nursing is the respect for life, dignity, and the rights of all persons. Nursing care is given a context mindful of the holistic nature of humans, understanding the body-mind-emotion-spirit. Nursing care is unrestricted by considerations of nationality, race, creed, color, age, sex, sexual preference, politics, or social status. Given that nurses practice in culturally diverse settings, professional nurses must have an understanding of the cultural background of clients in order to provide culturally appropriate interventions.

Nurses render services to clients who can be individuals, families, groups or communities. The client is an active participant in health care and should be included in all nursing care planning decisions.

To provide services to others, each nurse has a responsibility towards the client, co-workers, nursing practice, the profession of nursing, society, and the environment.

Nurses and Self

The nurse has a responsibility to model health care behaviors. Holistic nurses strive to achieve harmony in their own lives and assist others striving to do the same.

Nurses and the Client

The nurse's primary responsibility is to the client needing nursing care. The nurse strives to see the client as whole and provides care that is professionally appropriate and culturally consonant. The nurse holds in confidence all information obtained in professional practice and uses professional judgment in disclosing such information. The nurse enters into a relationship with the client that is guided by mutual respect and a desire for growth and development.

Nurse and Co-workers

The nurse maintains cooperative relationships with co-workers in nursing and other fields. Nurses have a responsibility to nurture each other and to assist nurses to work as a team in the interest of client care. If a client's care is endangered by a co-worker, the nurse must take appropriate action on behalf of the client.

Nurses and Nursing Practice

The nurse carries personal responsibility for practice and maintaining continued competence. Nurses have the right to use all appropriate nursing interventions and have the obligation to determine the efficacy and safety of all nursing actions. Wherever applicable, nurses use research findings in directing practice.

Nurses and the Profession

The nurse plays a role in determining and implementing desirable standards of nursing practice and education and research. Holistic nurses may assume a leadership position to guide the profession towards a holistic philosophy of practices. Nurses support nursing research and the development of holistically oriented nursing theories. The nurse participates in establishing and maintaining equitable social and economic working conditions in nursing.

Nurses and Society

The nurse, along with other citizens, has the responsibility for initiating and supporting actions to meet the health and social needs of all society..

Nurses and the Environment

Nurses strive to create a client environment to be one of peace, harmony, and nurturance so that healing may take place. The nurse considers the health of the ecosystem in relation to the need for health, safety, and peace of all persons.

Revised and re-approved by AHNA, 2007

POSITION ON NURSING RESEARCH AND SCHOLARSHIP

Holistic care refers to approaches and interventions that address the needs of the whole person: body, mind emotion and spirit focusing on healing the whole person as its goal. Nursing is the care and treatment of the human response to actual or potential health problems, concerns or life processes. Thus, nursing research and scholarship should assist its practitioners to : (1) understand the holistic nature of human experiences of health, healing and illness; and (2) evaluate the effects of holistic nursing actions on the client's health, healing, illness and recovery.

Research supporting holistic nursing includes descriptive, explanatory and exploratory designs that expand our understanding of holistic practice and enhances the evidence base for practice.

Holistic nursing research may be conducted using qualitative, quantitative, mixed methods or other approaches that further our understanding of phenomenon such as the complexity of the human condition, healing, and outcomes of holistic therapies. Research however, needs to be planned and results interpreted in a holistic, integral, or unitary framework for it to be considered "holistic" nursing research.

Several ways of knowing - rational/scientific, intuitive, and aesthetic — are recognized in holistic nursing research. Nursing scholarship involves intuitive and aesthetic approaches to comprehend the multi dimensional nature of our work which encompasses: (1) the art of care, (2) the wholeness of the client's experiences and meaning of patterns that emerge, (3) the beauty of authentic interaction; and (4) the knowledge of that which is perceived through non-verbal, non-objective expression. Nursing scholarship involves rational/empirical understanding that is necessary to demonstrate: (1) basic mechanisms of nursing actions and integrative therapies; (2) clinical safety, efficacy and treatment outcomes of holistic modalities; and (3) the interactive and integrative nature of body/mind/emotion/spirit.

Since many phenomena of concern to nursing remain unknown or undocumented such that exploratory, qualitative research is a highly effective method for expanding the disciplines' developing body of knowledge. Further, many aspects of the human responses to health, illness and life processes are subjective and qualitative research is the most feasible method of obtaining information and understanding of the human condition. In addition, sensitive measurement instruments that assess and document the interactive nature of each client's biological, psychological, emotional, sociological, and spiritual patterns are needed as well as ongoing evaluation of nursing interventions assessing their usefulness in promoting wellness and preventing illness.

The body of knowledge that frames holistic nursing includes knowledge of the science and understanding of the art of the profession. AHNA supports nursing research and scholarship that builds scientific knowledge through empirical work and that extends humanistic understanding through qualitative investigations and creative expressions. AHNA endorses and supports nursing scholarship relevant to learning, documenting and comprehending that which is the science and art of holistic nursing with the goal of producing dependable and relevant information to practitioners and the public.

Revised and re-approved by ANHA 2007

POSITION ON THE ROLE OF NURSES IN THE PRACTICE OF COMPLEMENTARY AND ALTERNATIVE THERAPIES

Overview

Complementary and alternative modalities (CAM) offer therapies that supplement conventional medical care. The National Center on Complementary and Alternative Medicine (NCCAM) of the National Institutes of Health has categorized five major domains of CAM practices:

- Whole Medical Systems, including acupuncture, Ayurveda, homeopathic medicine and naturopathic medicine

- Mind-Body Interventions, including meditation, certain uses of hypnosis, dance, music, art therapy and prayer

- Biologically-Based Therapies, including herbal, special dietary, orthomolecular, and individual biological therapies

- Manipulative and Body-Based Methods, including chiropracty and osteopathy

- Energy Therapies, including Qigong, Reiki, Healing Touch and Therapeutic Touch.

Holistic care refers to approaches and interventions that address the needs of the whole person: body, mind, emotion and spirit. Healing arts are those interventions that foster an individual's healing process, i.e., a return of the individual toward a state of wholeness in which body, mind, emotion, and spirit are integrated and balanced, and the person is able to reach deeper levels of personal understanding. Healing does not equate to curing, although they can be synchronous. The nursing profession has a long history of caring for individuals in a holistic manner and integrating the healing arts with conventional treatments. Florence Nightingale recognized the importance of caring for the whole person and encouraged interventions that enhanced individuals' abilities to draw upon their own healing powers. She considered touch, light, aromatics, empathetic listening, music, quiet reflection, and similar healing measures as essential ingredients to good nursing care. Today's education of registered nurses is built upon these same principles.

The American Holistic Nurses' Association (AHNA) is a professional nursing association dedicated to the promotion of holism and healing.

The AHNA believes that nurses enter therapeutic partnerships with clients, their families, and their communities to serve as facilitators in the healing process. The holistic caring process supported by AHNA is one in which nurses:

- Acquire and maintain current knowledge and competency in holistic nursing practice, including CAM therapies and practices integrated within that practice
- Provide care and guidance to persons through nursing interventions and therapies consistent with research findings and other sound evidence
- Hold to a professional code of ethics and healing that seeks to preserve wholeness and dignity of self and others
- Engage in self-care and further develop their own personal awareness of being an instrument of healing
- Recognize each person as a whole: body-mind-spirit
- Assess clients holistically, using appropriate traditional and holistic methods
- Create a plan of care in collaboration with the clients and their significant others consistent with cultural background, health beliefs, sexual orientation, values, and preferences that focuses on health promotion, recovery or restoration, or peaceful dying so that the person is as independent as possible

Nursing and CAM

The AHNA believes that inherent in the nursing role is the ability to assess, plan, intervene, evaluate, and perform preventive, supportive, and restorative functions of the physical, emotional, mental, and spiritual domains. Therefore, it is expected that the nurse may draw upon and utilize principles and techniques of both conventional and CAM therapies, and that these would be within the scope of nursing practice. AHNA supports the integration of CAM into conventional health care to enable the client to benefit from the best of all treatments available. In their provision of holistic care, nurses employ practices and therapies from both CAM and conventional medicine.

Consistent with conventional nursing practice, nurses must be competent in the CAM therapies and practices they use. The AHNA believes nurses integrate these practices into conventional care as part of a holistic practice. In addition, nurses support and assist clients with their use of CAM provided by other practitioners by:

- Identifying the need for CAM interventions,
- Assisting clients in locating providers of CAM interventions
- Facilitating the use of CAM interventions through education, counseling, coaching, and other forms of assistance
- Coordinating the use of CAM among various health care providers involved in clients' care; and evaluating the effectiveness of clients' complete integrative care

AHNA's Position

The AHNA believes that although selected CAM are appropriate interventions for use by nurses, the use of these interventions must be integrated into a comprehensive holistic nursing practice. Practicing within a holistic nursing framework does not imply competency in effectively and safely utilizing CAM therapies and practices. Nurses must be responsible for seeking, when necessary, additional education and experience and demonstrating clinical competency in all interventions used in their nursing practice.

A nurse practicing as a therapist of a specific conventional or CAM therapy, must have the education, skills, and credentials ascribed for that therapy. The nurse also must operate within the legal scope of practice of the nurse's licensure and jurisdiction.

AHNA views nurses as being in a unique position in the implementation of CAM throughout the health care system in that registered nurses:

- represent the greatest number of health care professionals, representing more than 2.7 million health care professionals, and are employed in more diverse clinical settings than any other health care professional;
- are uniquely prepared to differentiate normality from illness, provide interventions for health promotion and illness-related care, and use a wide range of medical technology and the healing arts;

- are advocates for clients rather than specific products or practices, therefore are in an excellent position to assure appropriate and adequate use of all types of services; and
- are trusted and held in high esteem by consumers.

These factors support nurses holding a leadership role in the implementation of CAM in various service settings and the coordination of CAM utilization by clients as part of an integrated approach to care.

Revised and re-approved by AHNA February 2007.

INDEX

Pages from *Standards of Holistic Nursing Practice* (2005; reproduced in Appendix B) and *Standards of Advanced Practice Holistic Nursing Practice for Graduate-Prepared Nurses* (2005; reproduced in Appendix C) are indicated by brackets [ ].

A

Access, 33–34
Advanced practice holistic nursing, 20, [99]
   assessment, 40, [110]
   collaboration, 58
   collegiality, 57
   communication, [107–108]
   consultation, 50
   coordination of care, 47
   cultural competence, [109–110]
   data collection and, 39, 41, 45, 52, 55
   diagnosis or health issues, 41
   education, 20, 21, 51, [104]
   ethics, 60, [102–103]
   evaluation, 52, [113]
   health teaching and health promotion, 49
   implementation, 46, [111–112]
   leadership, 65–66
   outcomes identification, 43, [111]
   planning, 45, [111]
   prescriptive authority and treatment, 51
   professional practice evaluation, 56
   quality of practice, 54
   reimbursement, 33
   research, 32, 62, [104–106]
   resource utilization, 63
   self-care, [106–107]
   standards (development), xii–xiii
   standards (previous), [93–117]
   See also Basic level of holistic nursing practice; Holistic nursing
Advocacy, 8, 20, 23, 37
   ethics and, 59
Age-appropriate care. *See* Cultural competence

Allopathic/conventional therapies. *See* Conventional/allopathic therapies
Alternative medical systems. *See* Whole medical systems
American Holistic Nurses Association (AHNA), 3–5, 19, 20, 21–22
   certification and continuing education by, 21–22, 27
   development of standards, x–xiv
   position statements, 59, 119
American Nurses Association (ANA)
   Code of Ethics for Nurses with Interpretive Statements, ix, 3, 10, 59
   Nursing: Scope and Standards of Practice, ix, 3
   Nursing's Social Policy Statement, ix, 3
Analysis. *See* Critical thinking, analysis, and synthesis
Art and science of holistic nursing. *See* Core values of holistic nursing
Assessment, 11, 39–40
   Standard of practice, 40, [90, 110]

B

Barriers to use, 33–34
Basic level of holistic nursing practice
   assessment, 39, [90]
   collaboration, 58
   collegiality, 57
   collaboration, 58
   communication, [89]
   coordination of care, 47
   cultural competence, [89]
   defined, 1–3
   diagnosis or health issues, 41
   education, 55, [87]
   ethics, 59–60, [102–103]
   evaluation, 52, [91]

Basic level of holistic nursing practice
(*continued*)
   health teaching and health promotion, 48
   implementation, 46
   leadership, 64
   outcomes identification, 42, [89]
   planning, 44–45, [90–91]
   professional practice evaluation, 56
   quality of practice, 53–54
   research, 61, [87]
   resource utilization, 63
   roles, 7–8, 37
   self-care, [88]
   standards (development), x
   standards (previous), [86–91]
   work environment, 17–18
   See also Advanced practice holistic nursing; Holistic nursing
Biologically based therapies, 12, 79, 124
   See also Complementary/alternative modalties (CAM)
Bioelectromagnetic-based therapies, 79
   See also Complementary/alternative modalties (CAM)
Biofield therapies, 79
   See also Complementary/alternative modalties (CAM)
Body of knowledge, 2, 9, 14–15, 16, 20, 30, 31, 33, 34
   assessment and, 39
   collaboration and, 58
   collegiality and, 57
   education and, 55
   implementation and, 46
   leadership and, 64, 65
   planning and, 45
   prescriptive authority and treatment, 51
   quality of practice and, 53
   research and, 62

C

CAM therapies. *See* Complementary/alternative modalities
Care recipient. *See* Patient
Care standards. *See* Standards of practice

Caring process, 10–13, 38
Case management. *See* Coordination of care
Certification and credentialing, 21–22, 27, 31
   defined, 22
   education and, 19, 31
   reimbursement and, 33
   requirements, 22
Chronic conditions, 24, 28
Client. *See* Patient
Clinical practice, 32–33
Clinical settings. *See* Practice settings
Code of Ethics for Holistic Nurses, [102–103], 120
Code of Ethics for Nurses with Interpretive Statements, ix, 3, 10, 59
   See also Ethics
Collaboration, 15, 37, 58
   See also Healthcare providers; Interdisciplinary health care
Collegiality, 57
Commitment to the profession, 22–23
Communication, 14–16, [89]
   See also Holistic communication
Competency, 31–32
   See also Certification and credentialing
Complementary/alternative modalities (CAM), 27–30
   benefits, 25–26
   categories, 79–80
   defined, 67
   position (AHNA) on, 124–127
   use, 25, 28, 30
Community resources and systems, 21, 46, 47, 60, 63
Consultation, 16, 18, 50
Continuity of care, 42, 58
Context, 14
Conventional/allopathic therapies and interventions, 2, 7, 11–16 *passim*, 25–30 *passim*, 37, 58, 59
   defined, 67
Coordination of care, 47, 64
   See also Interdisciplinary health care
Core values of holistic nursing, 8–17, [85–91, 100–113]

Phenomenon of concern, 2, 122
Planning, 38
  collaboration and, 58
  resource utilization and, 63
  standard of practice, 44–45, [90–91, 111]
Policy. *See* Healthcare policy
Practice as holistic nursing principle, 7, 36
Practice environment, 5, 15, 17–18
  collegiality and, 57
  quality of practice, 54
  therapeutic practice standard, [89, 108–109]
Practice roles. *See* Roles in holistic nursing practice
Practice settings. *See* Practice environment
Practice standards. *See* Standards of Practice
Prescriptive authority and treatment standard of practice, 51
Presence, 1, 8, 13, 14, 15, 32, 36
  defined, 70
Prevention, 29
Principles of holistic nursing, 6–8, 35–38
Process. *See* Nursing process
Professional development
  collegiality and, 57
  education and, 20, 23
  See also Education; Leadership
Professional organizations, 23
  See also American Nurses Association
Professional performance. *See* Standards of professional performance
Professional practice evaluation
  standard of professional performance, 56

Q

Quality of practice
  standard of professional performance, 53

R

Recipient of care. *See* Family; Patient
Referrals. *See* Collaboration; Coordination of care
Registered Nurse, 18–22
  assessment and, 39–40
  collaboration, 58
  collegiality, 57
  consultation, 50
  coordination of care, 47
  diagnosis or health issues, 41
  education, 55
  ethics, 59–60
  evaluation, 52
  health teaching and health promotion, 48–49
  implementation, 46
  leadership, 64–66
  outcomes identification, 42–43
  planning, 44–45
  prescriptive authority and treatment, 51
  professional practice evaluation, 56
  quality of practice, 53–54
  research, 61–62
  resource utilization, 63
Regulatory issues. *See* Laws, statutes, and regulations
Reimbursement, 33
Relationship-centered care
  defined, 70
Research, 2, 4, 5, 7, 8, 11, 16–17, 32
  collaboration and, 58
  core value of, 16–17, [87], [104–106]
  position (AHNA) on, 122–123
  standard of practice, [87], [104–106]
  standard of professional performance, 61–62
  See also Evidence-based practice
Resource utilization
  standard of professional performance, 63
Roles in holistic nursing practice, 7–8, 37
  See also Registered Nurse